Having a Baby

Kathryn Hollins, Anna Cox, Milli Miller, Tessa van der Vord and Scott Watkin

illustrated by Beth Webb

series editor Sheila Hollins

Beyond Words

herhead

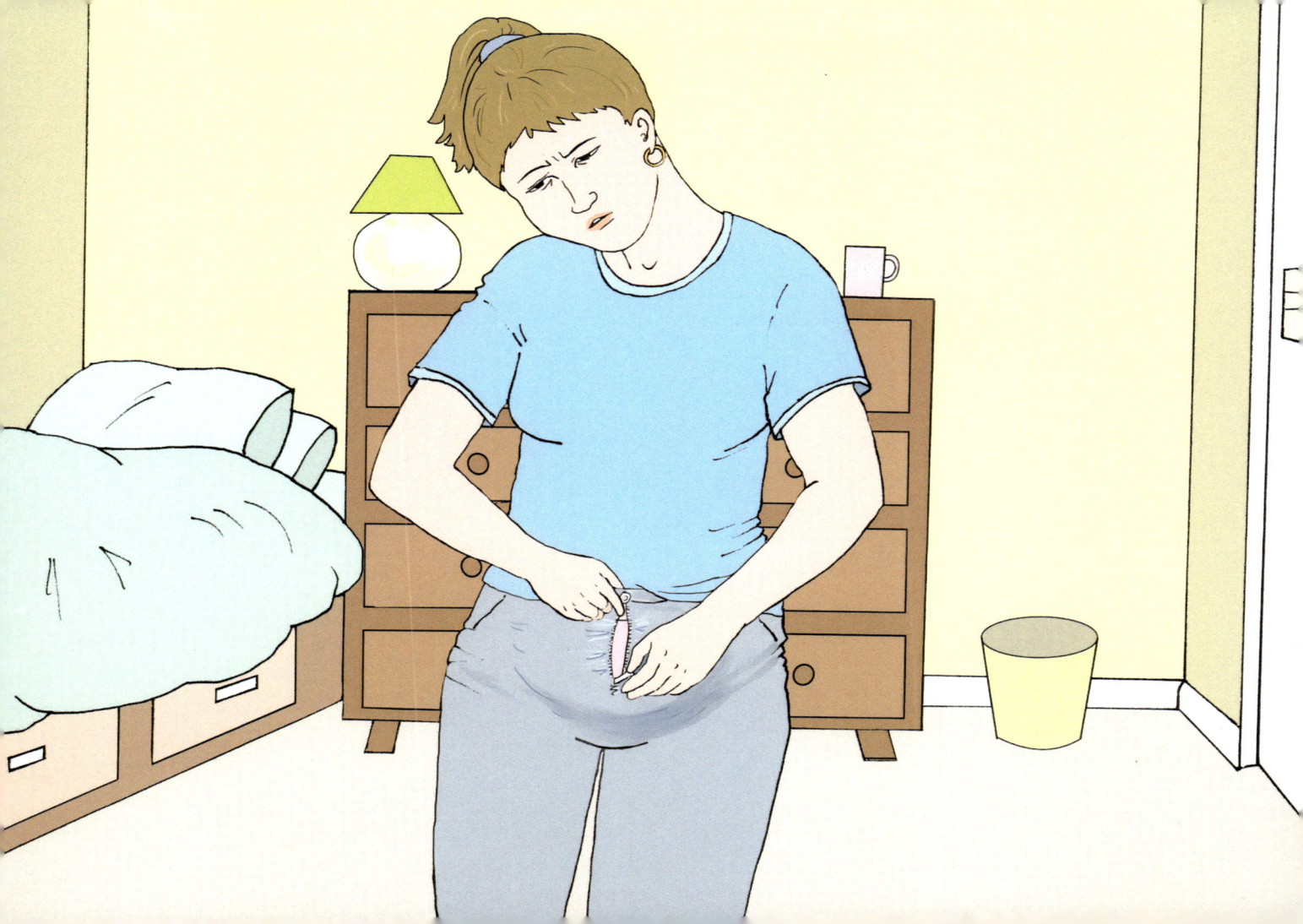

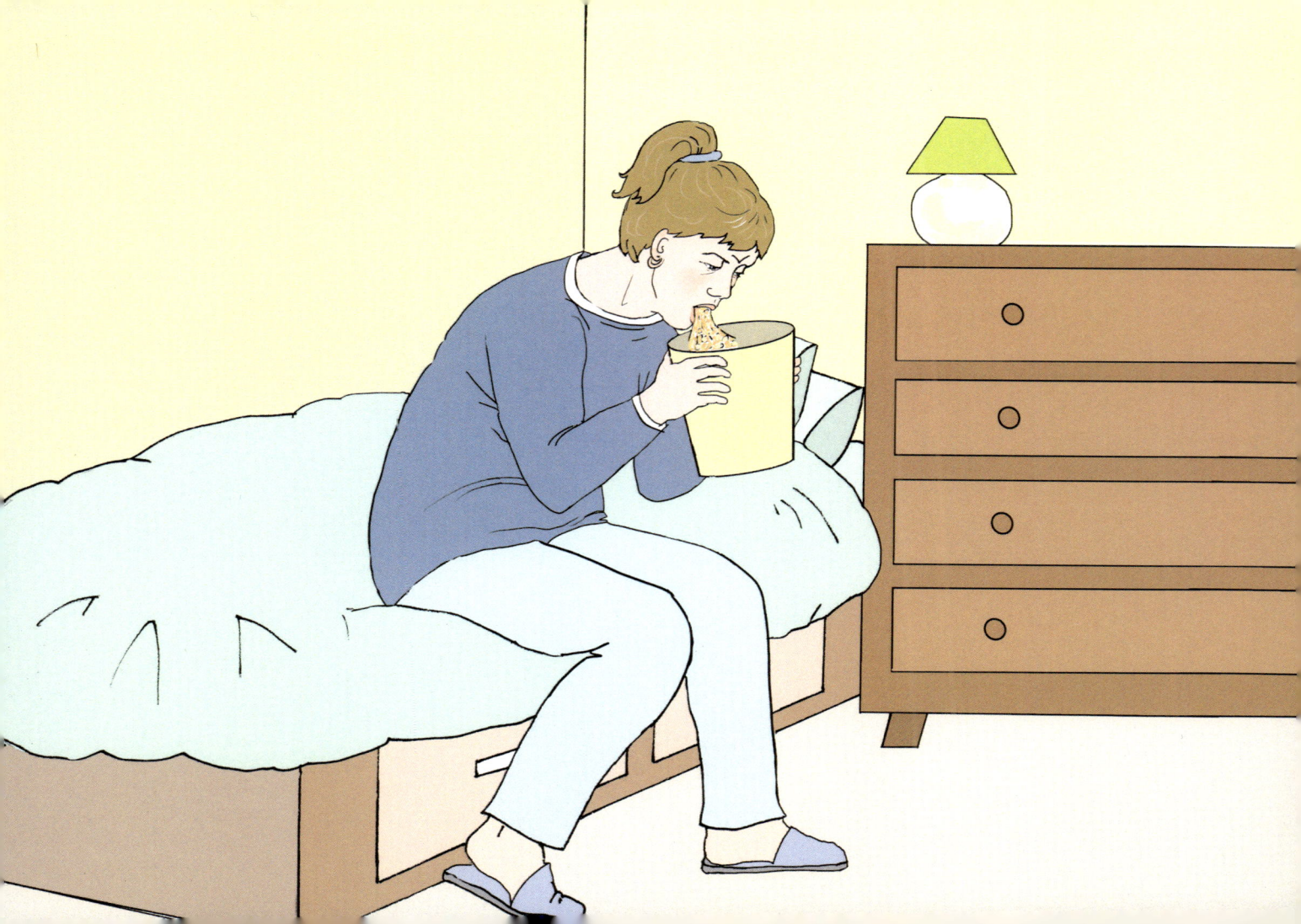

3

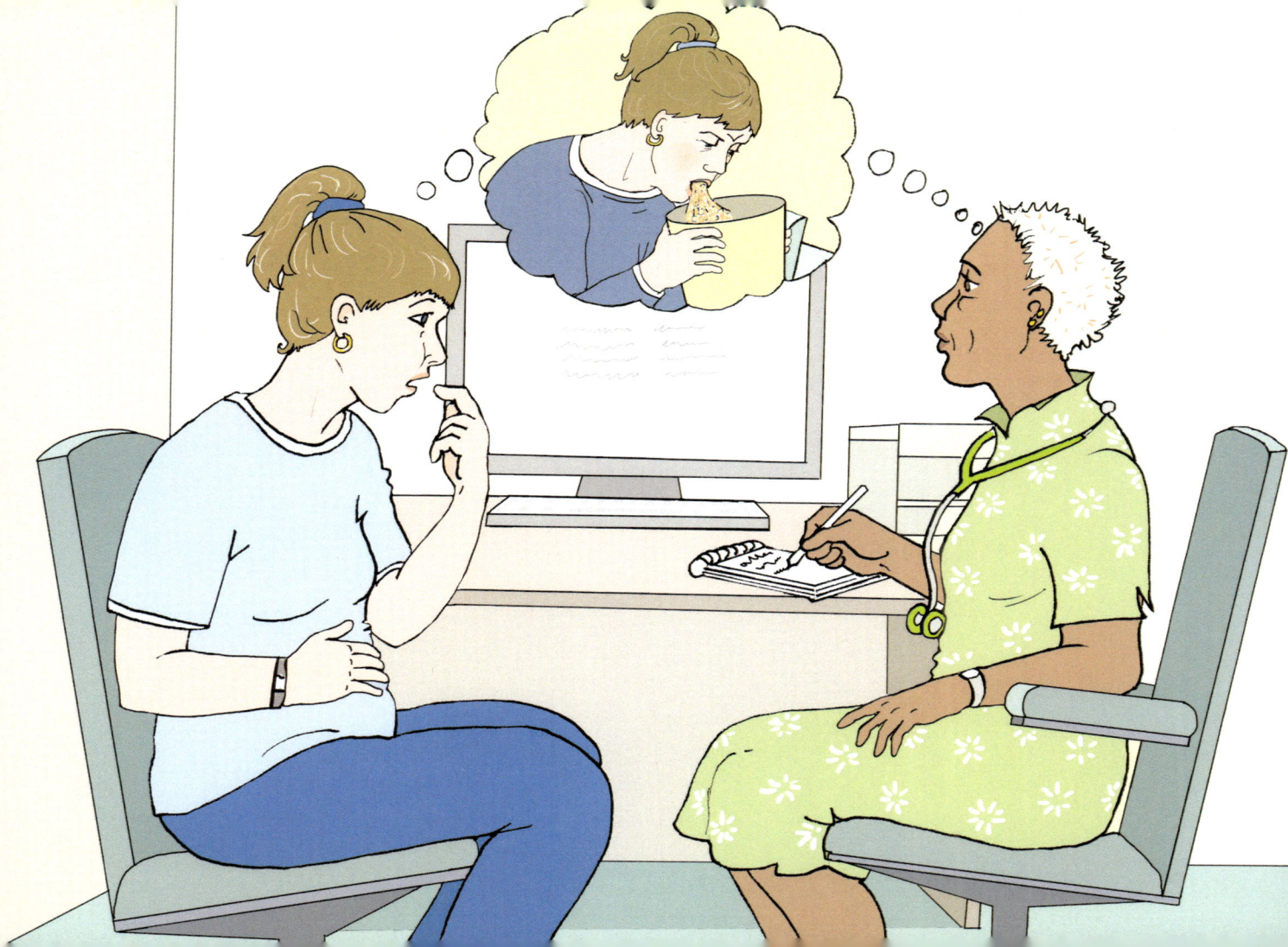

4

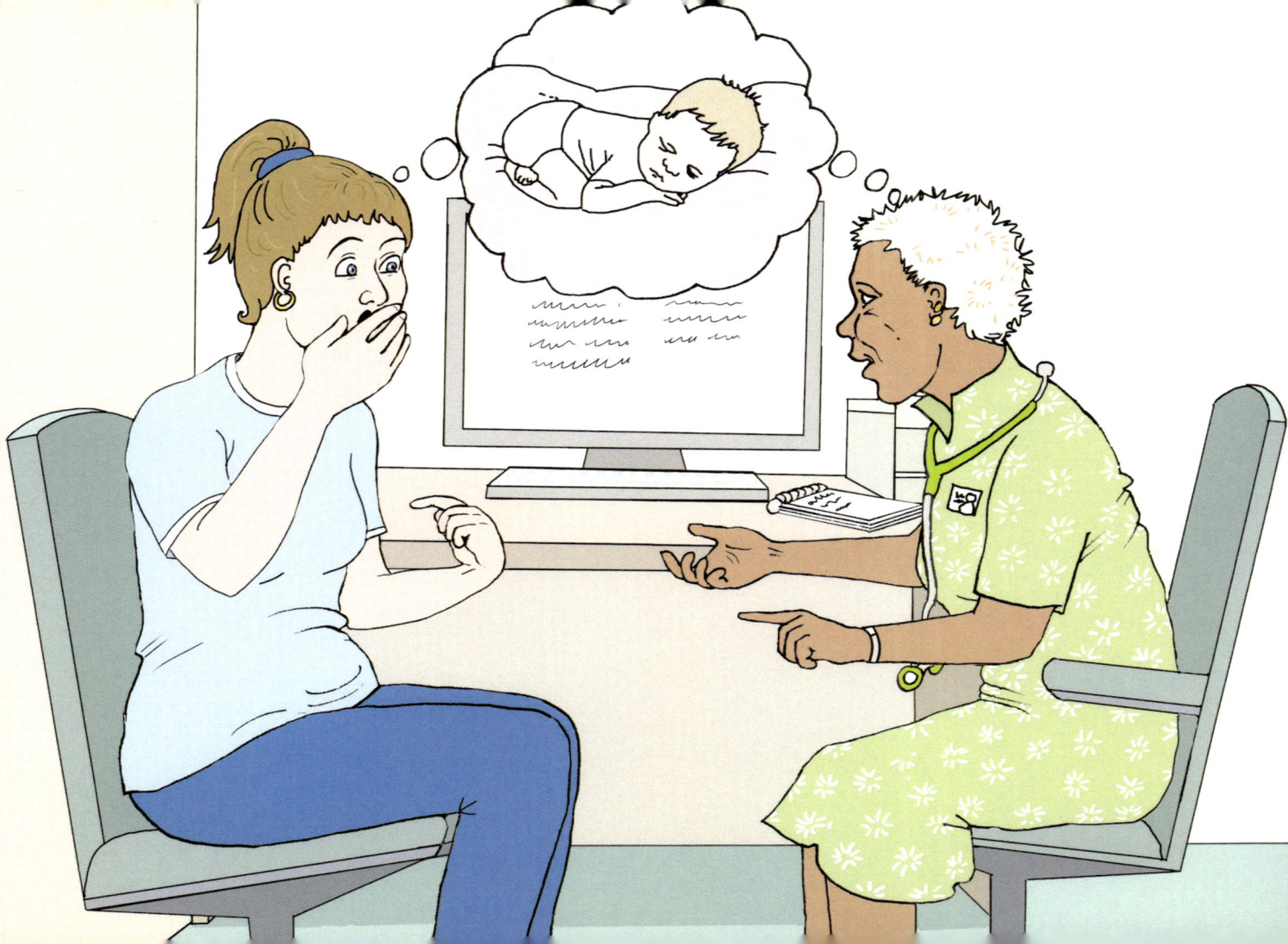

5

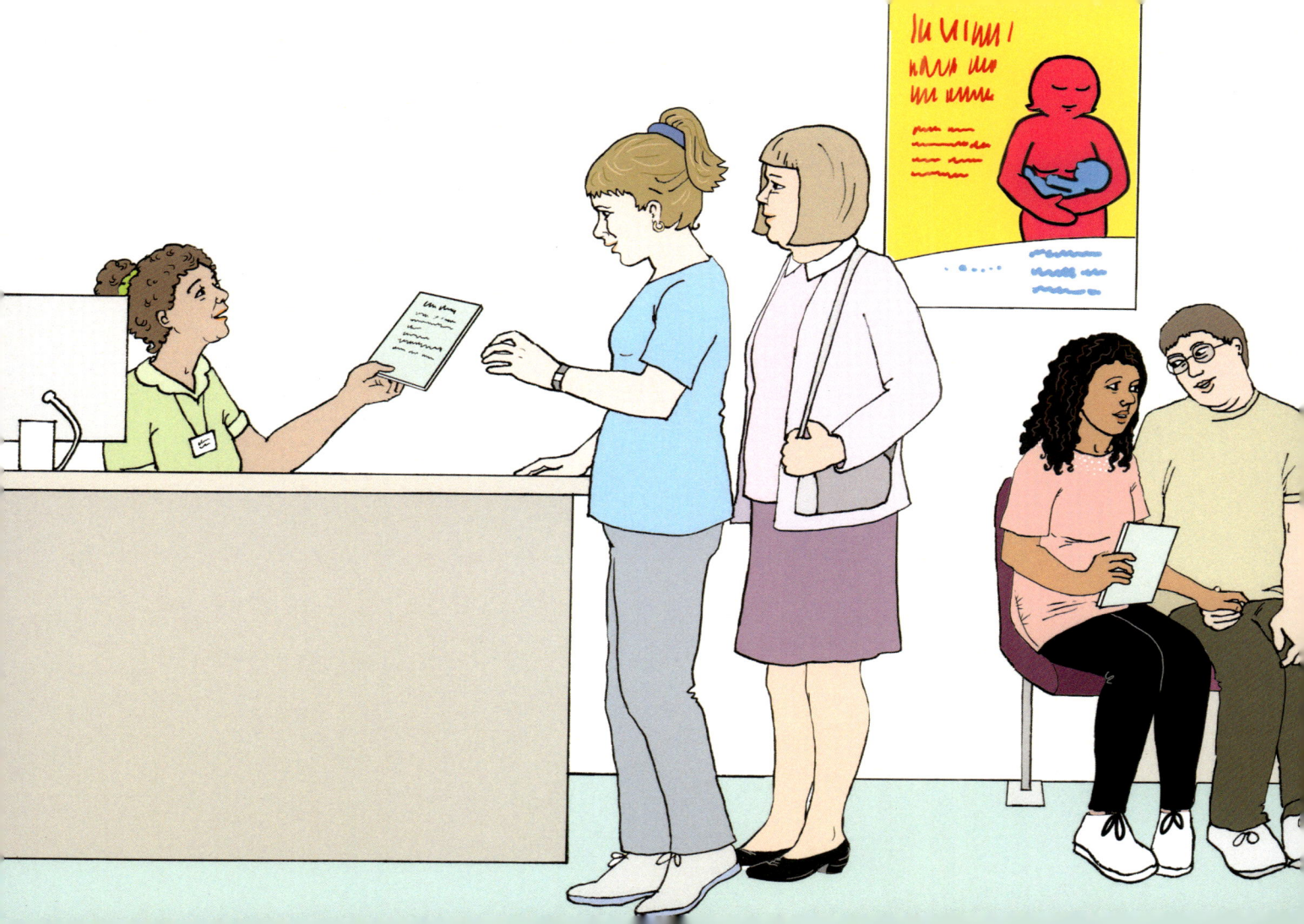

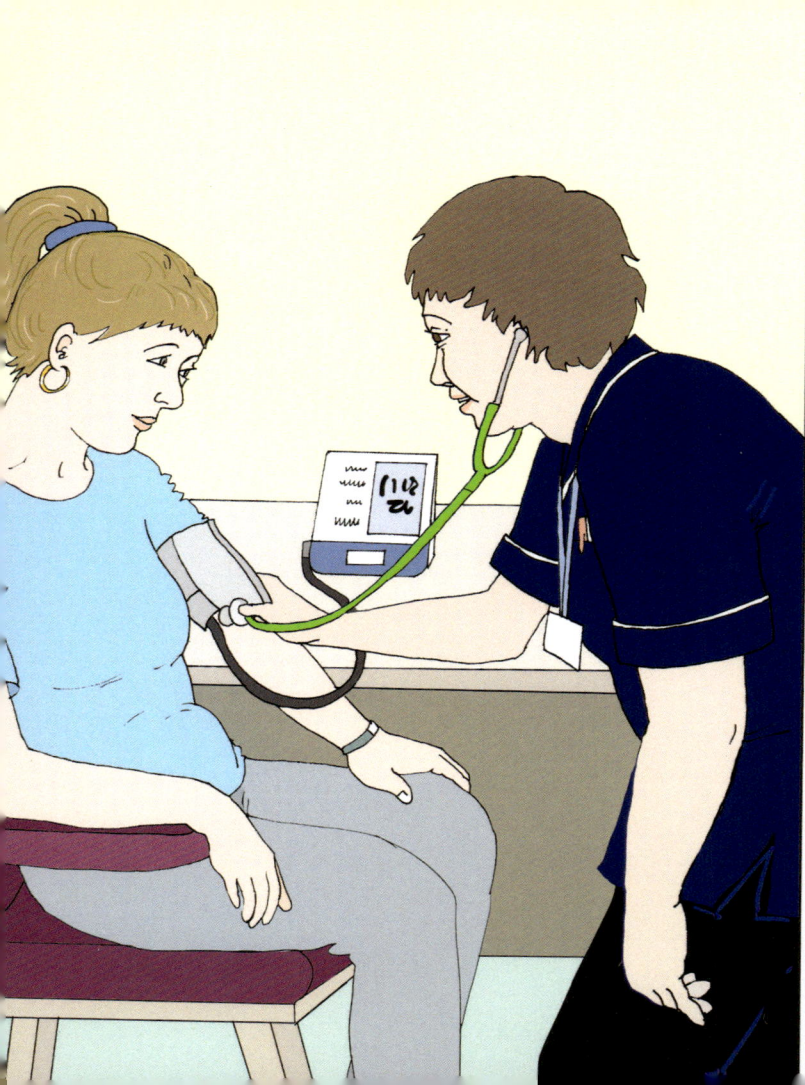

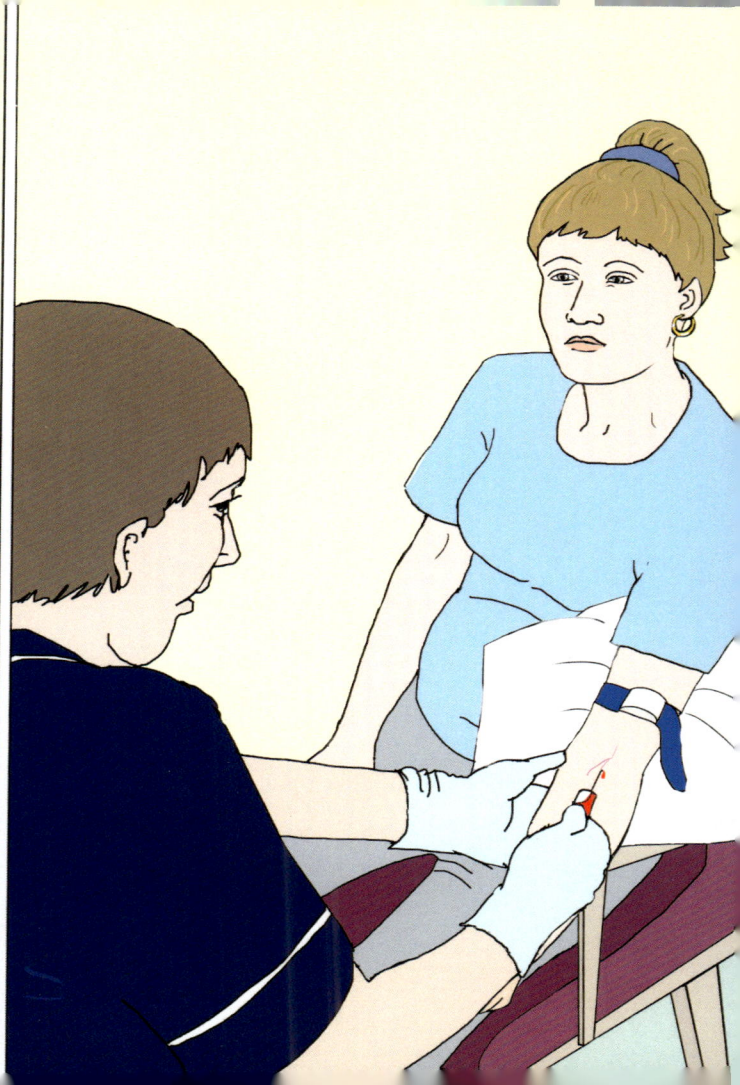

7

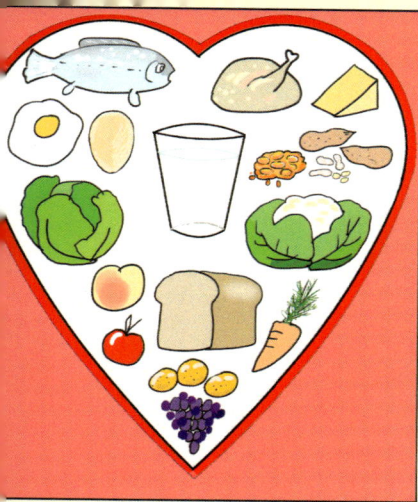

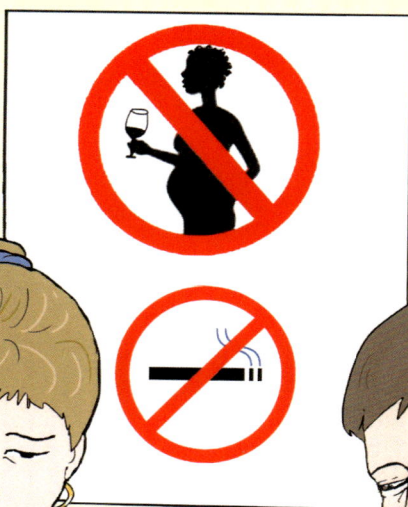

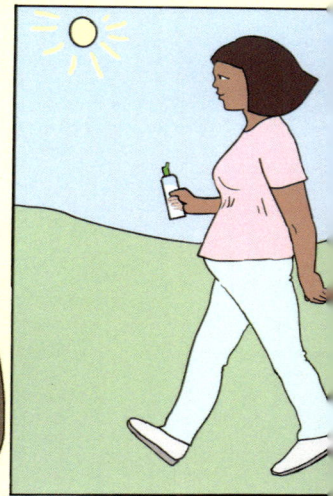

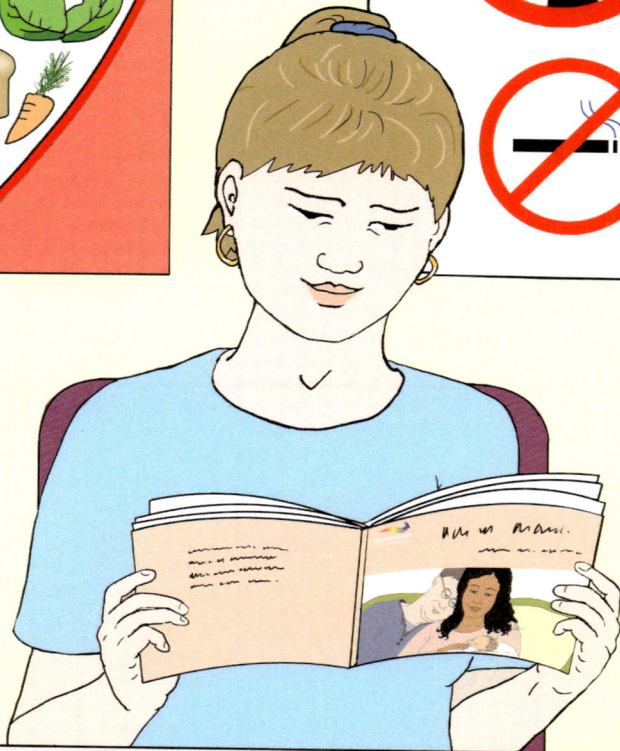

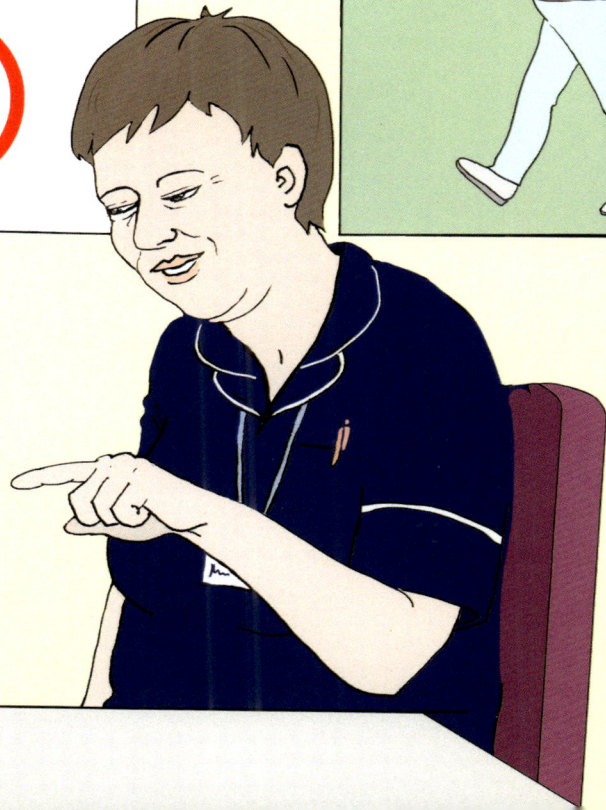

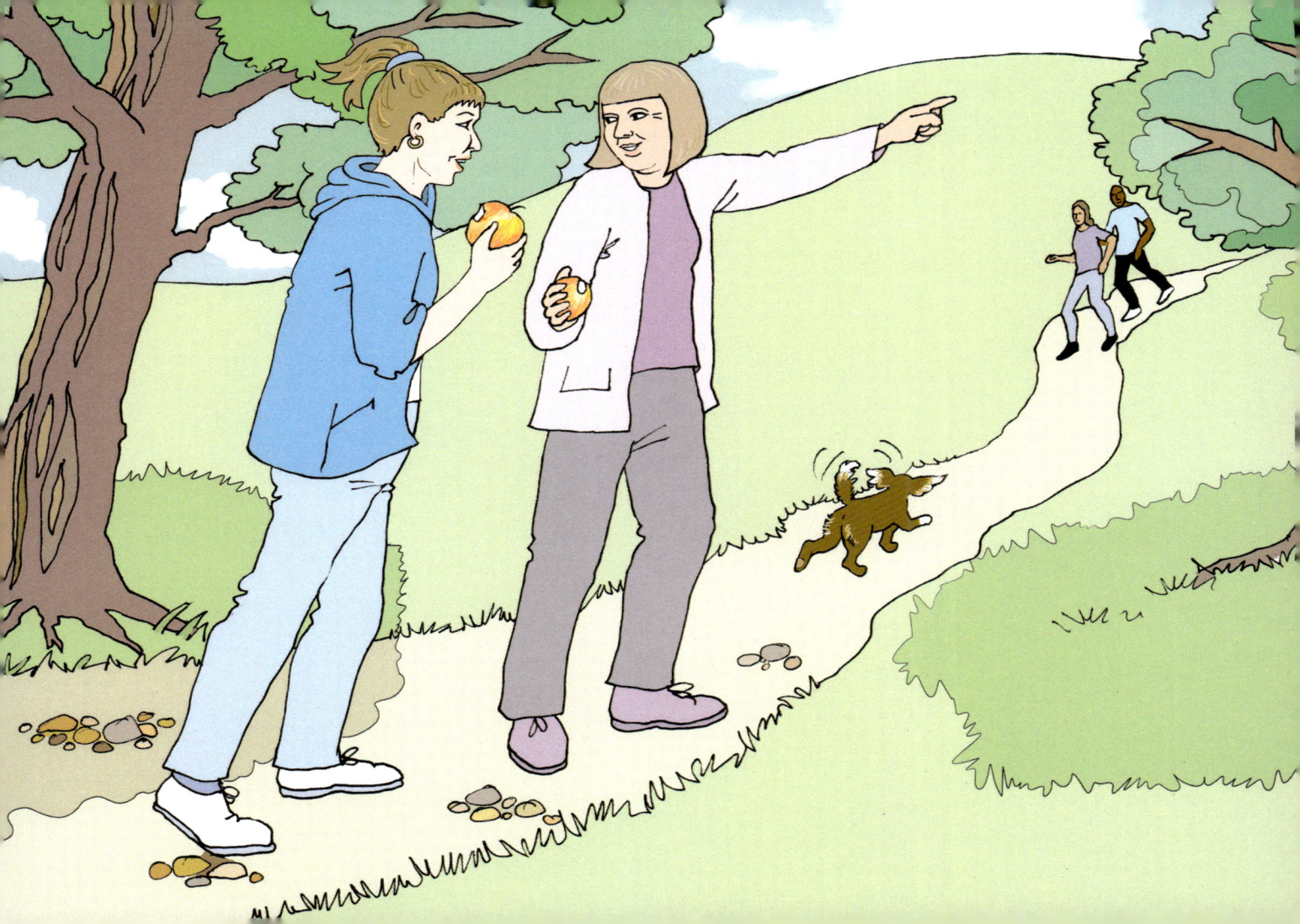

9

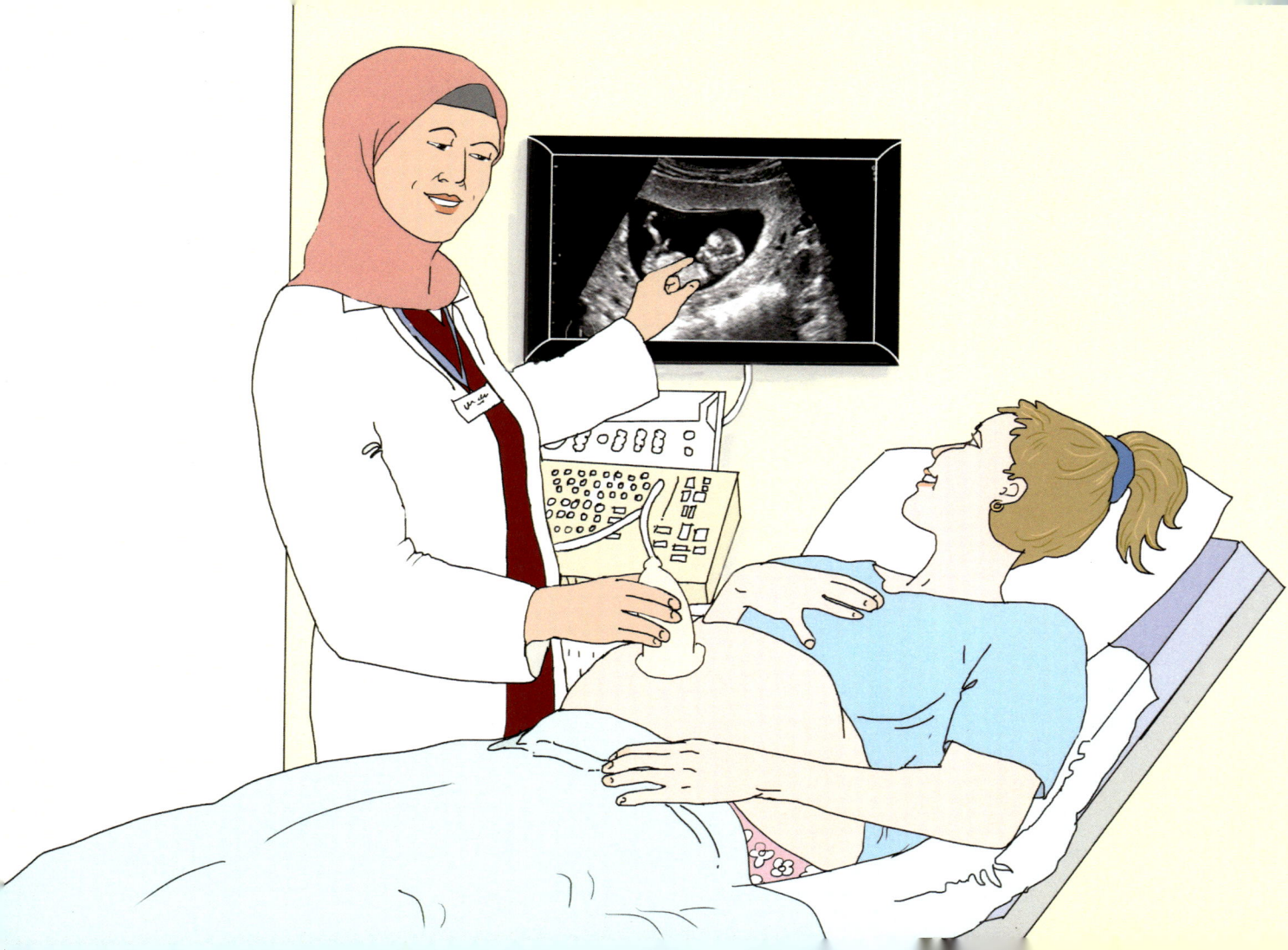

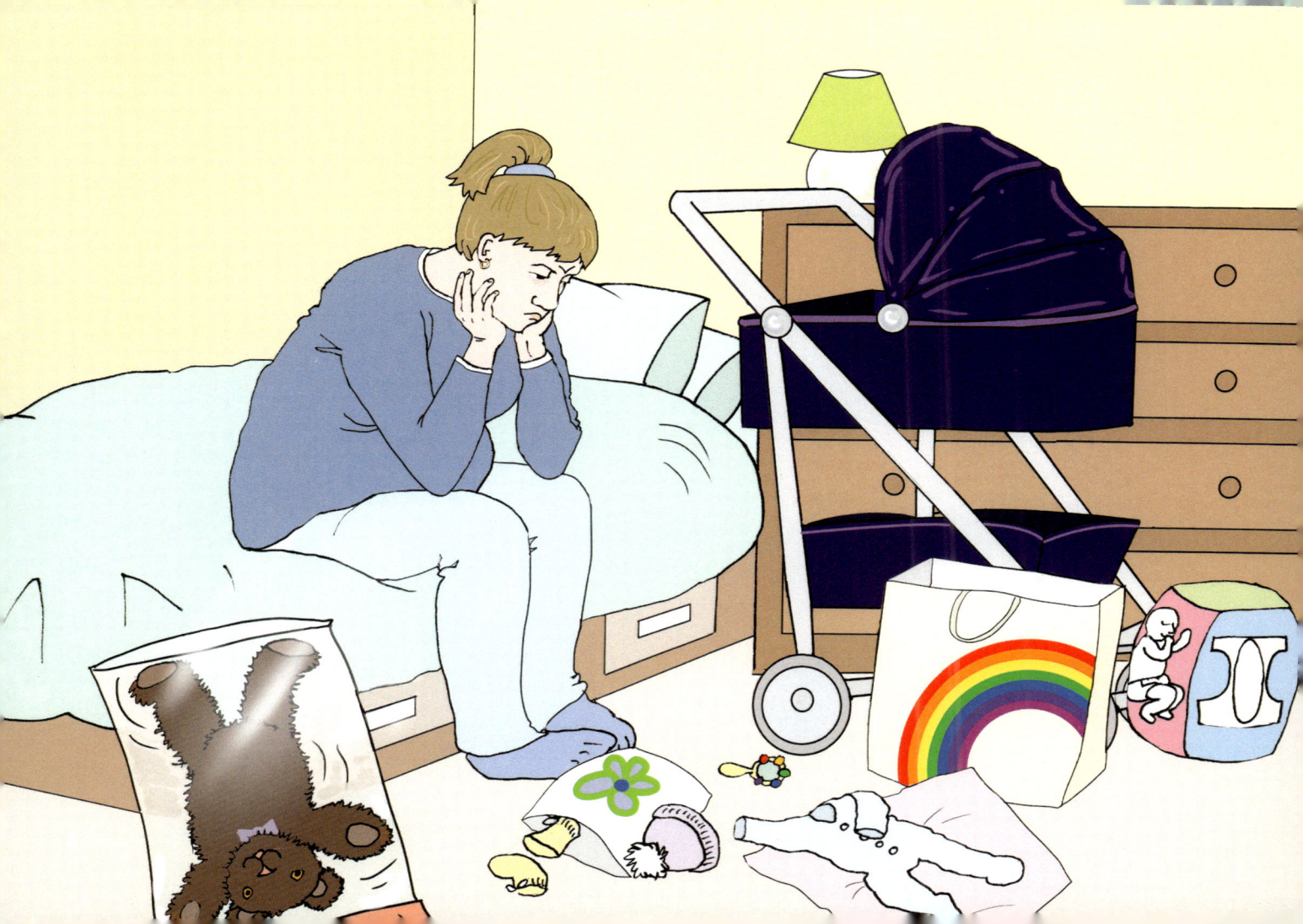

11

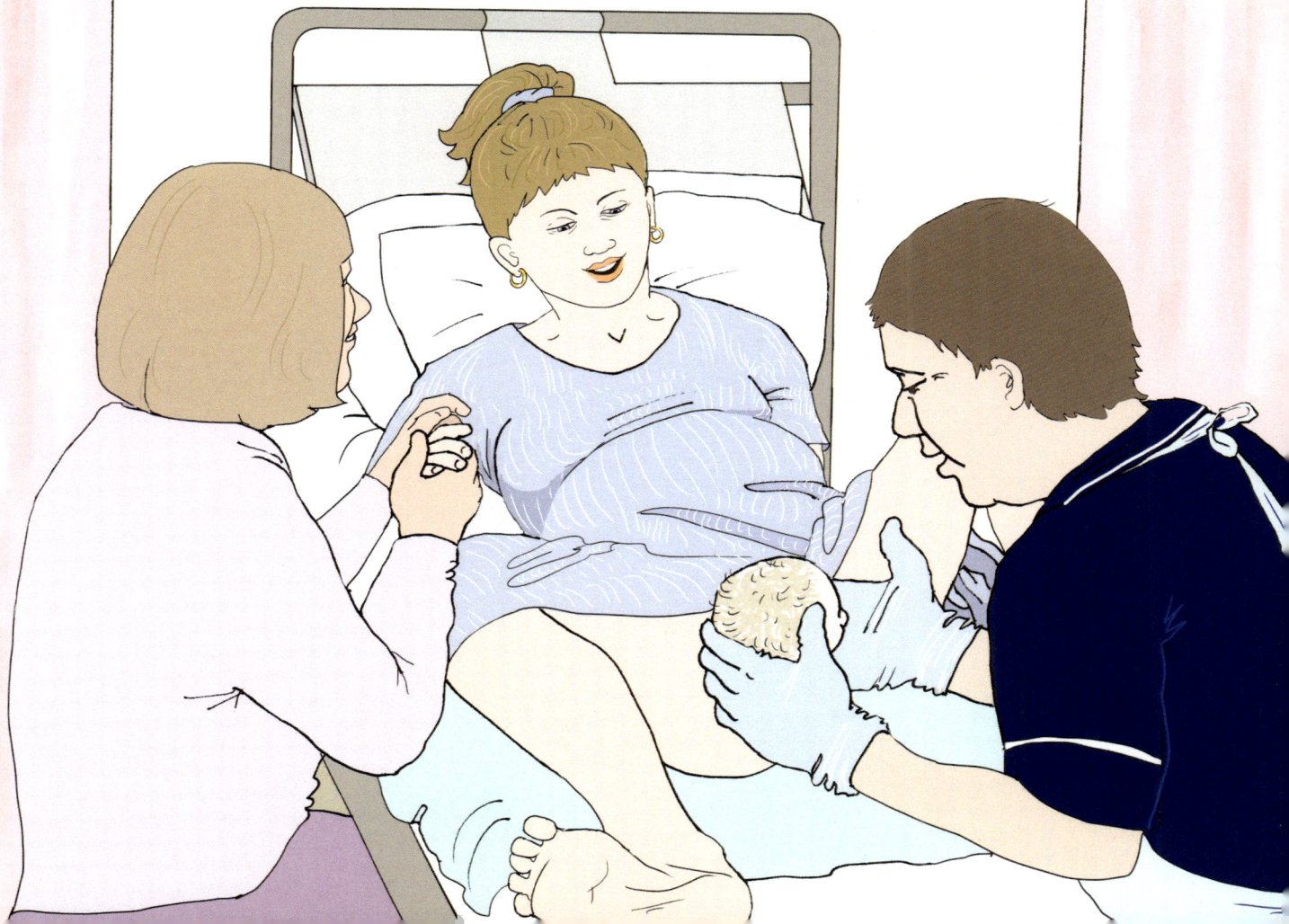

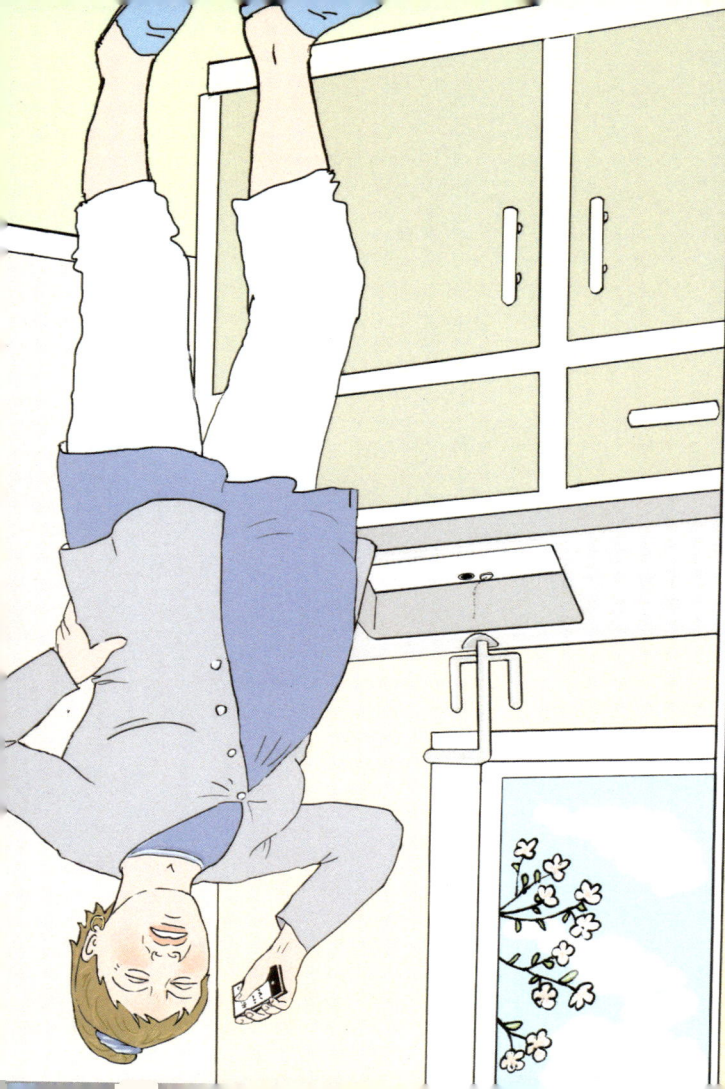

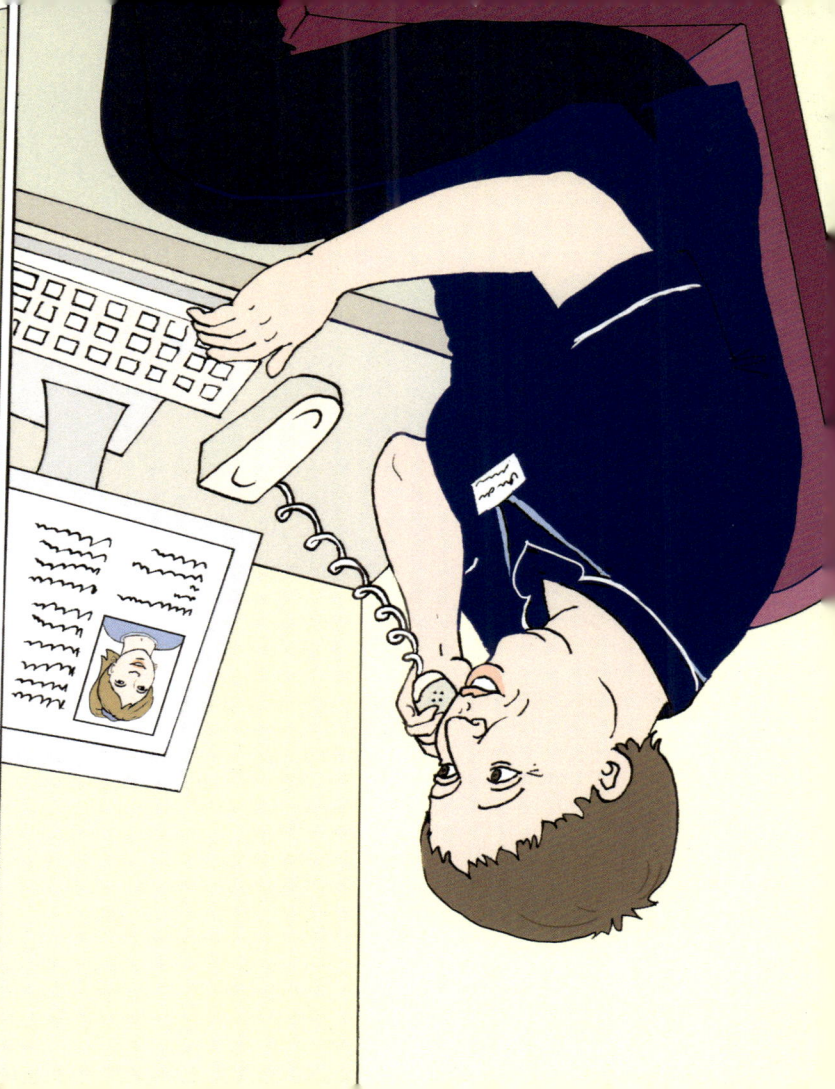

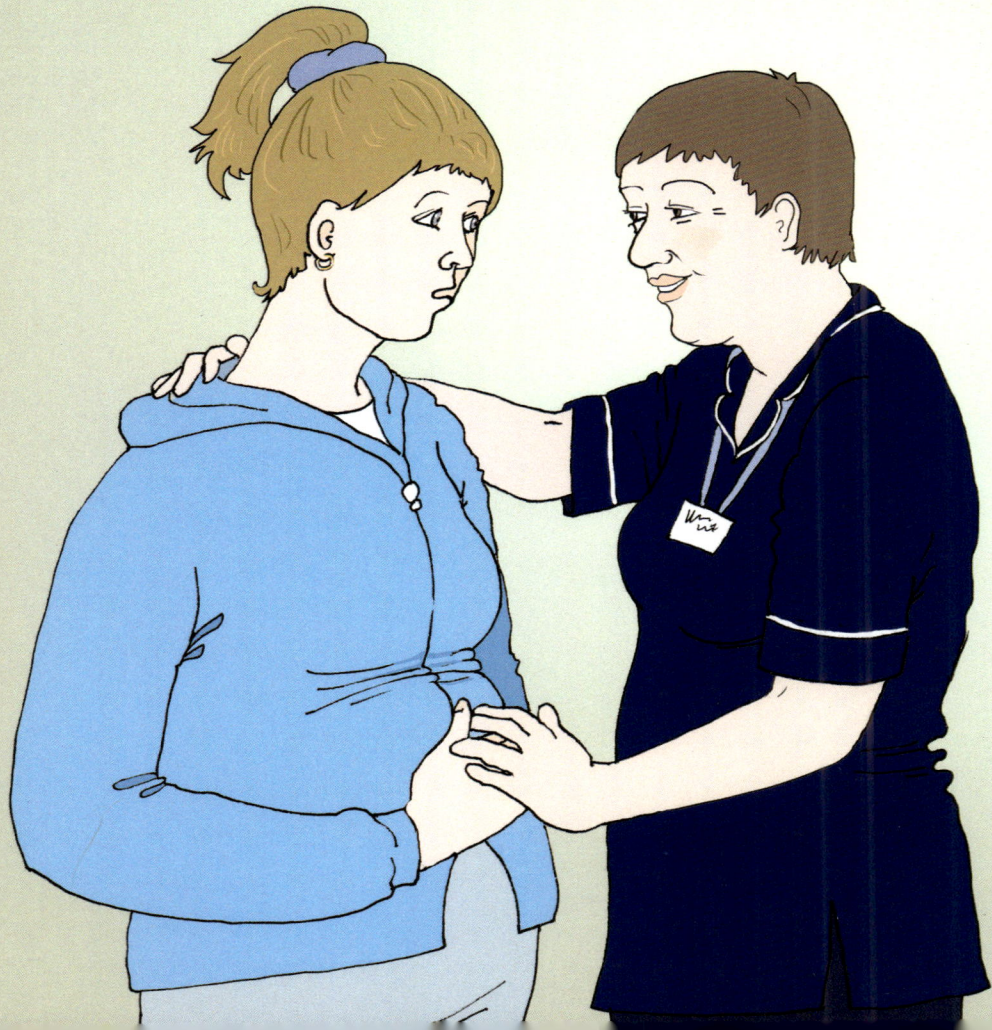

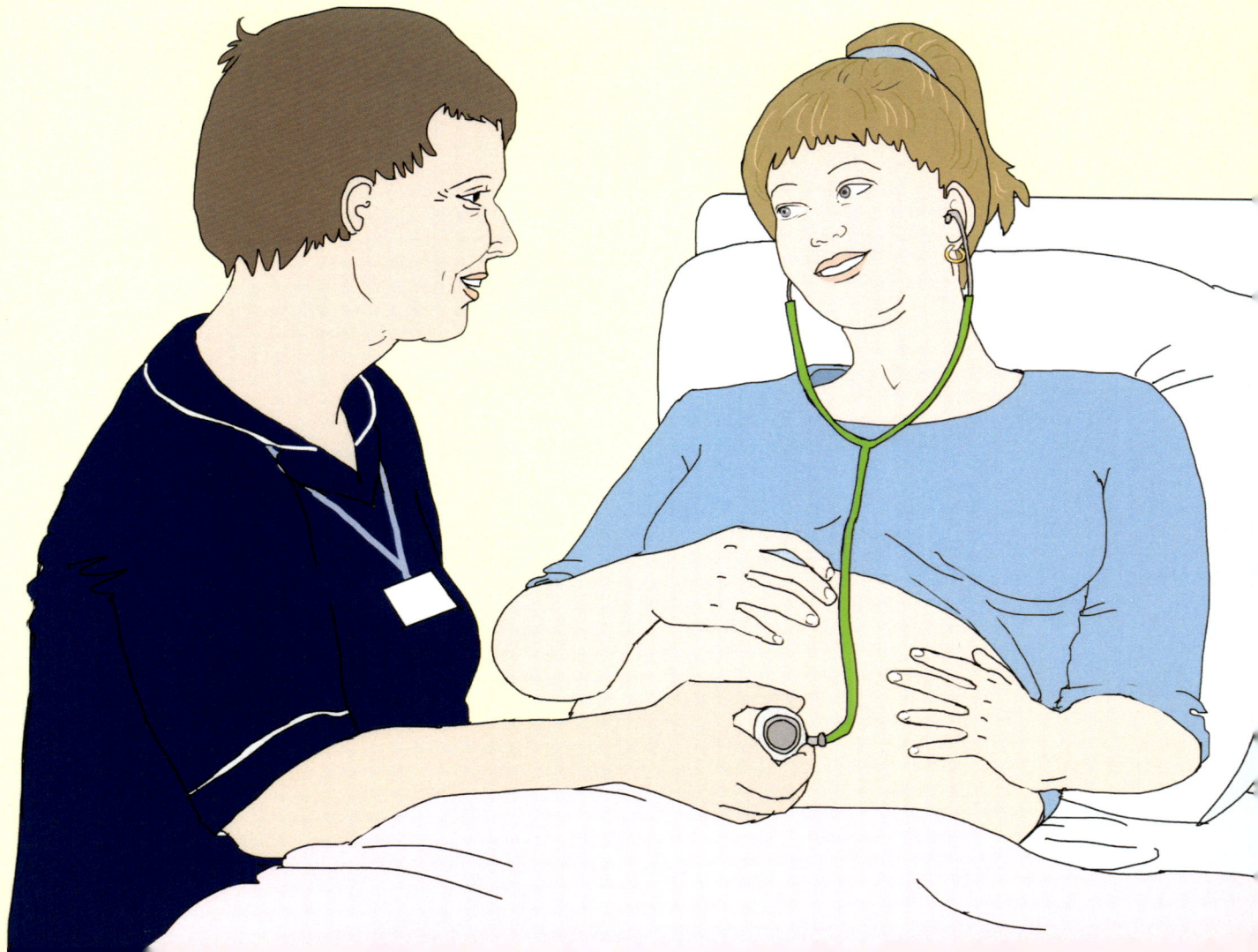

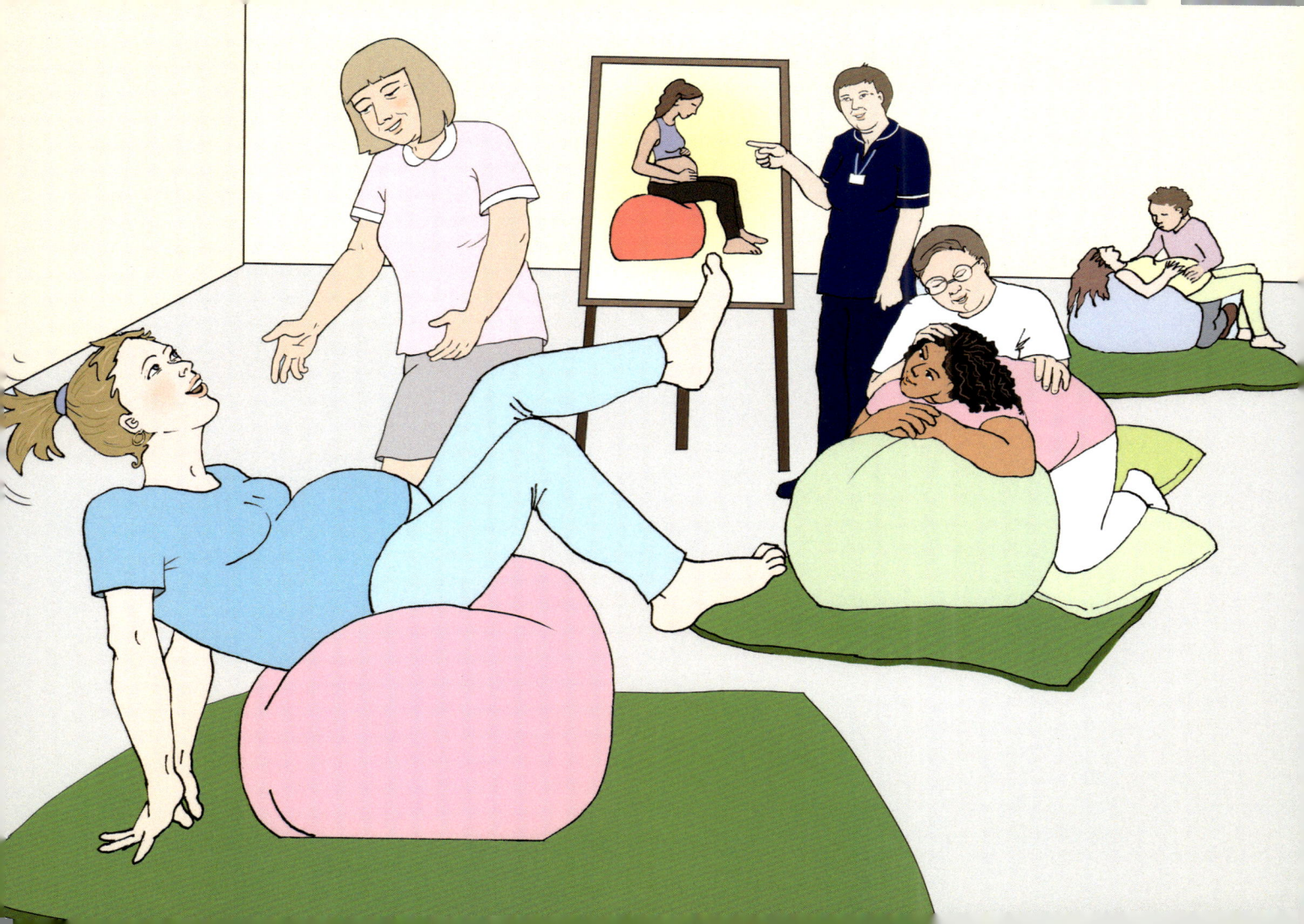

14

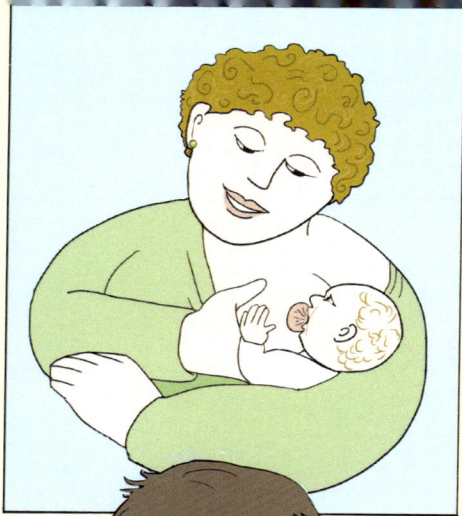

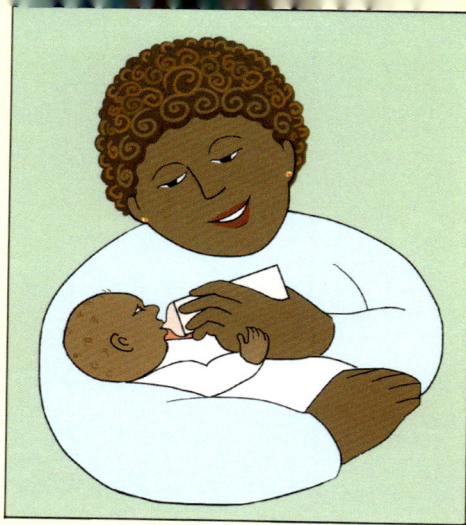

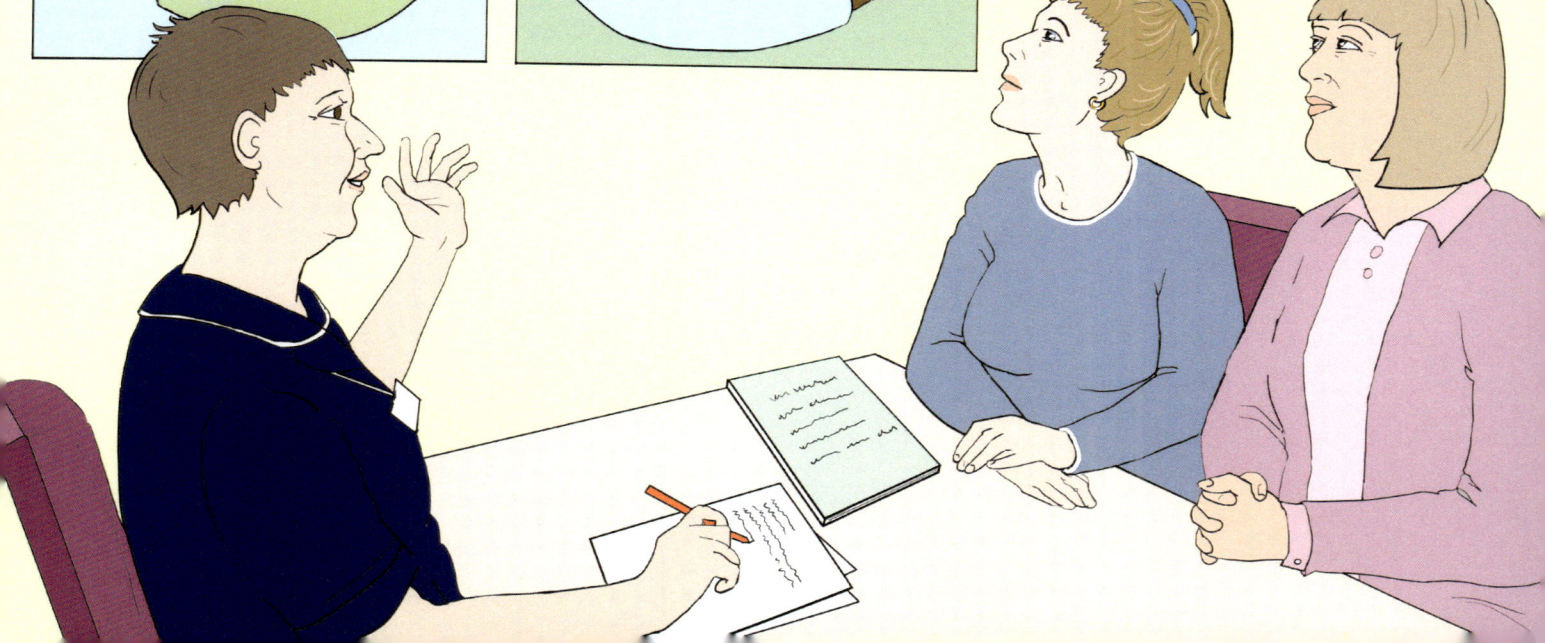

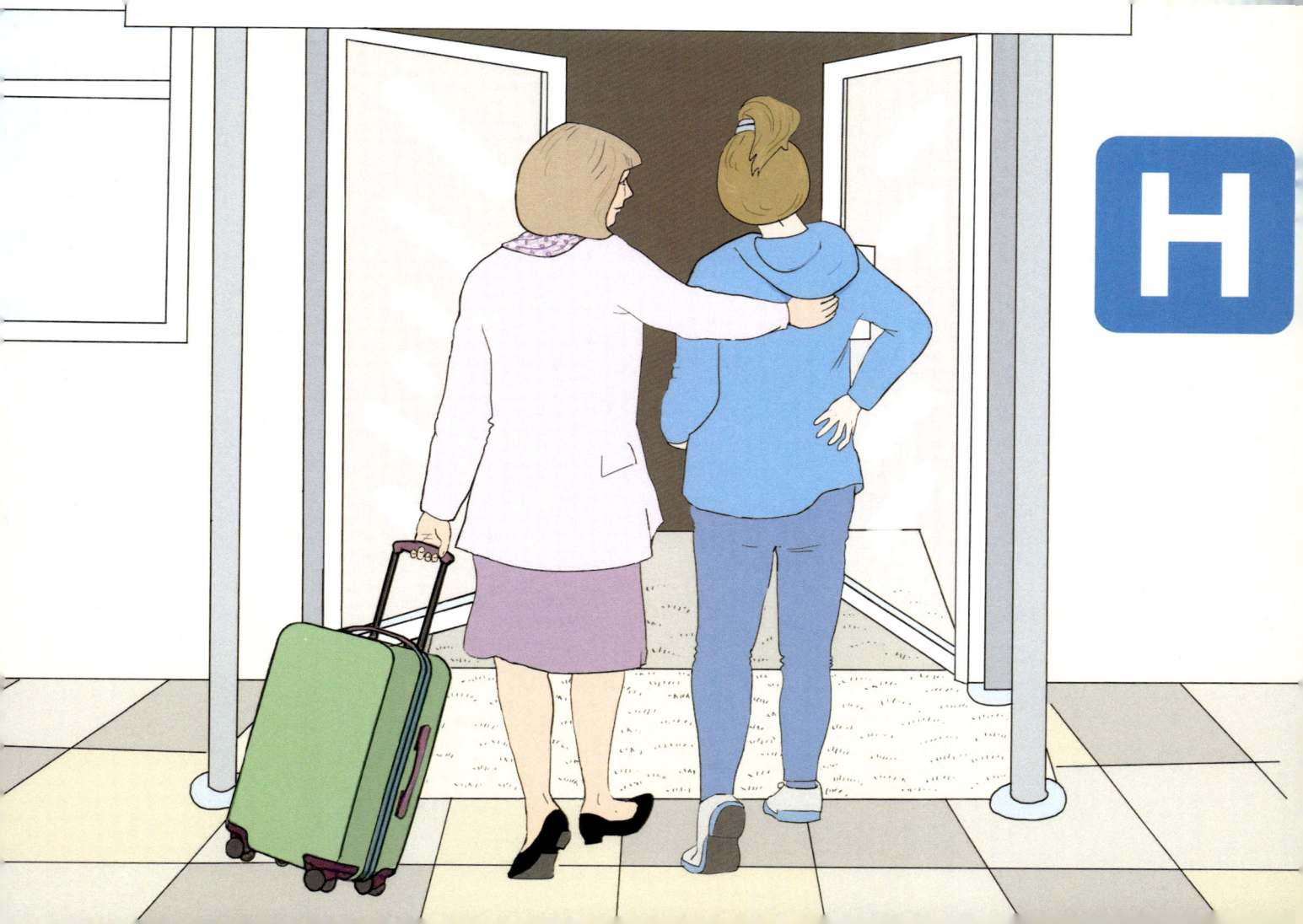

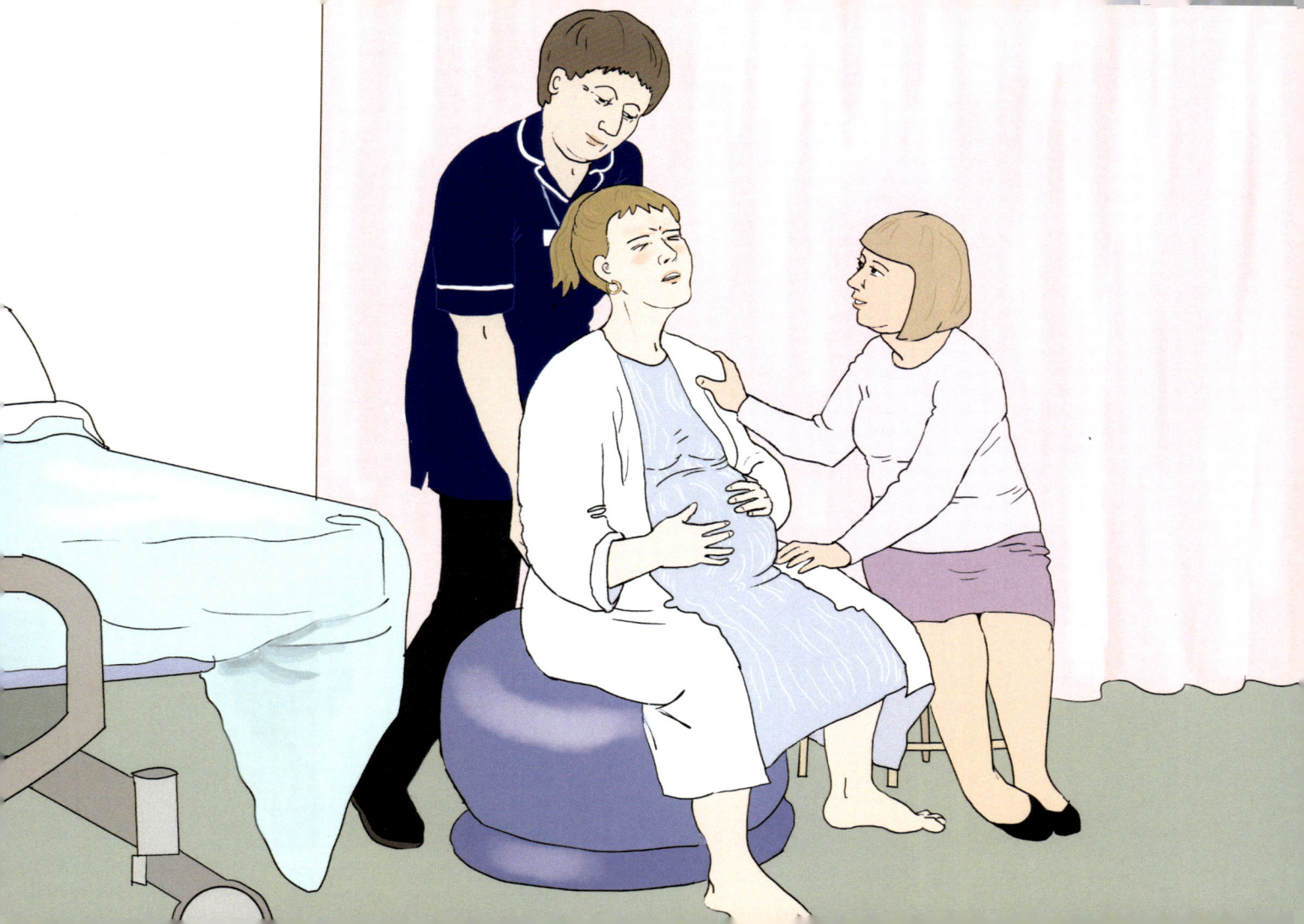

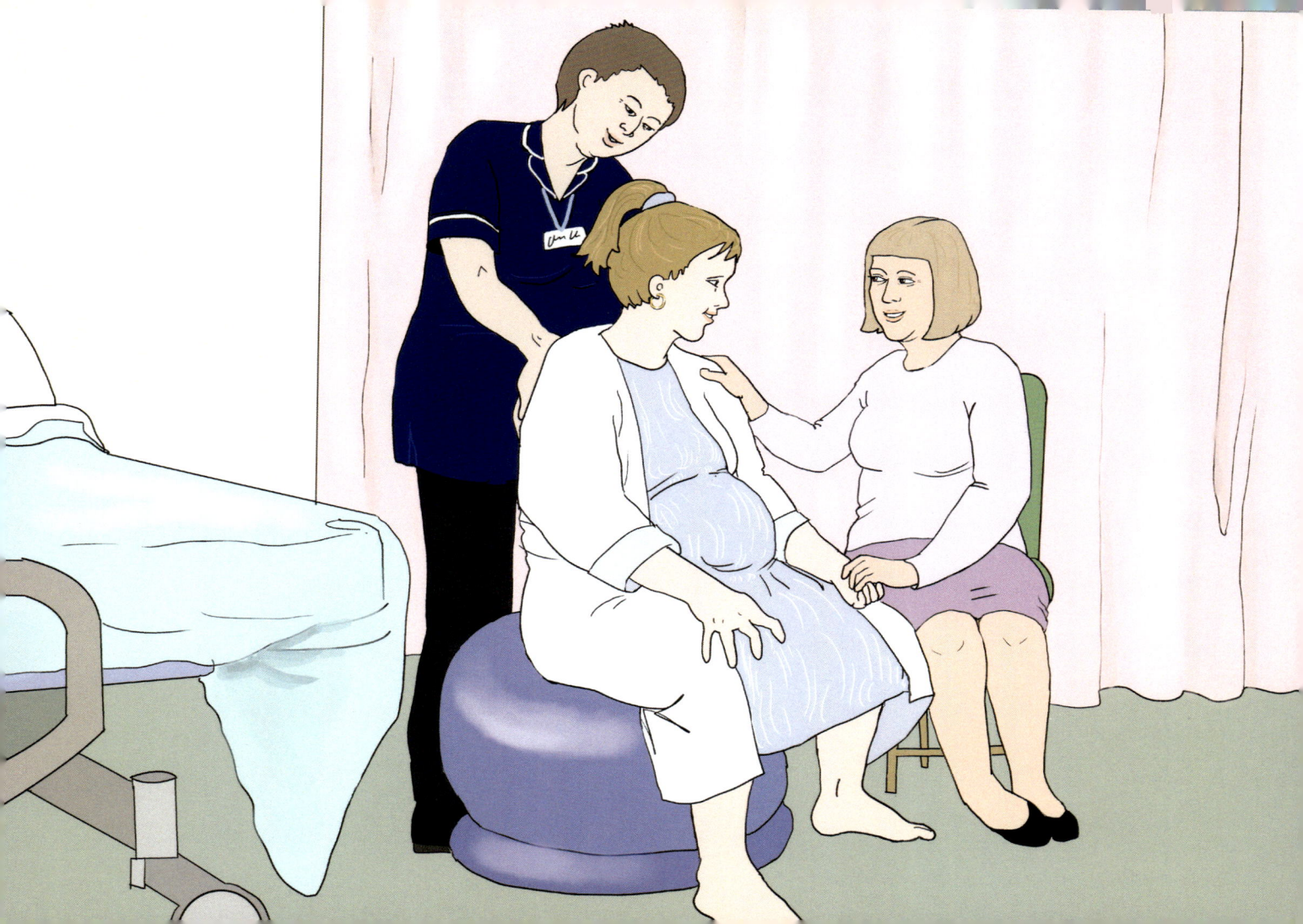

19

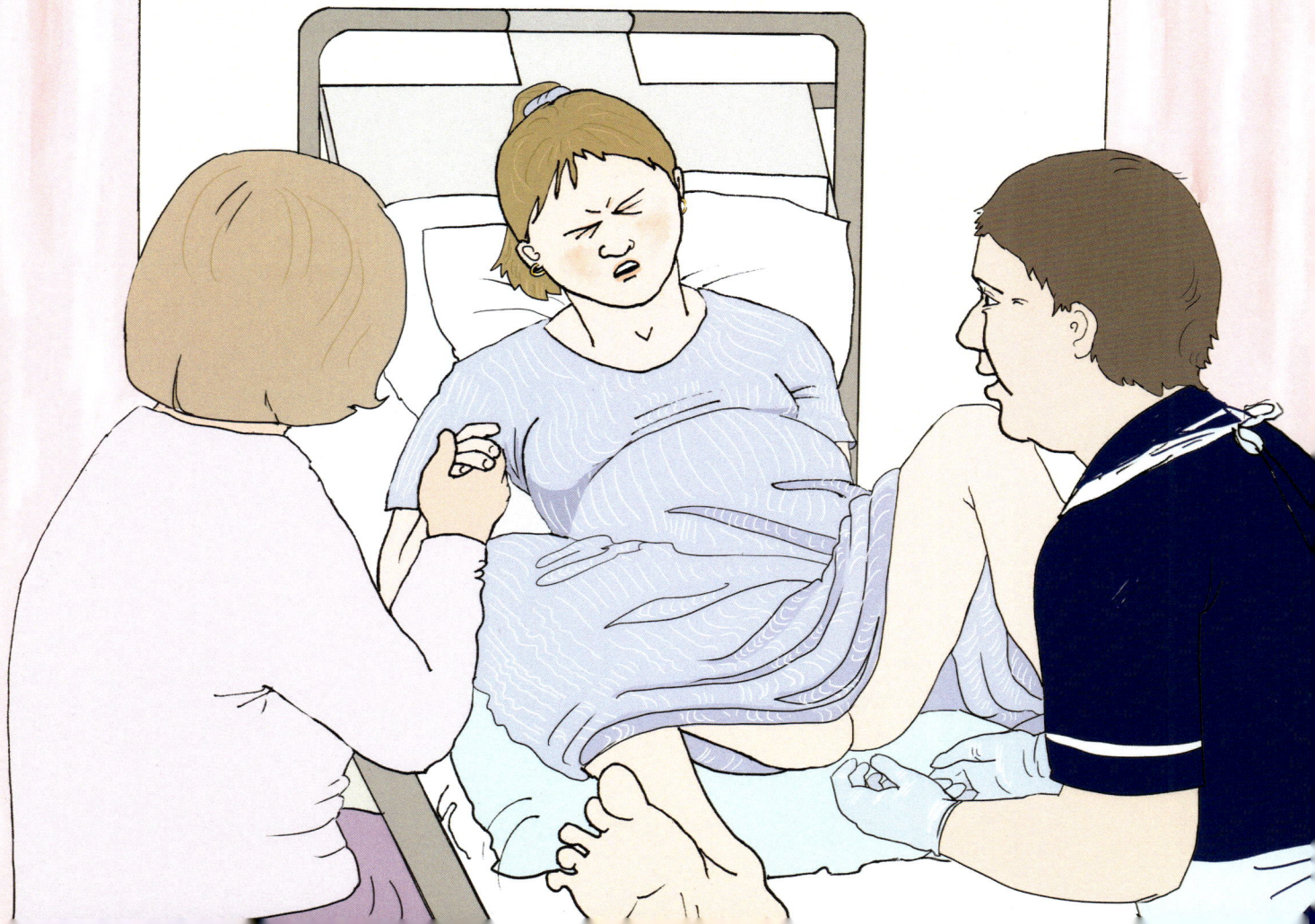

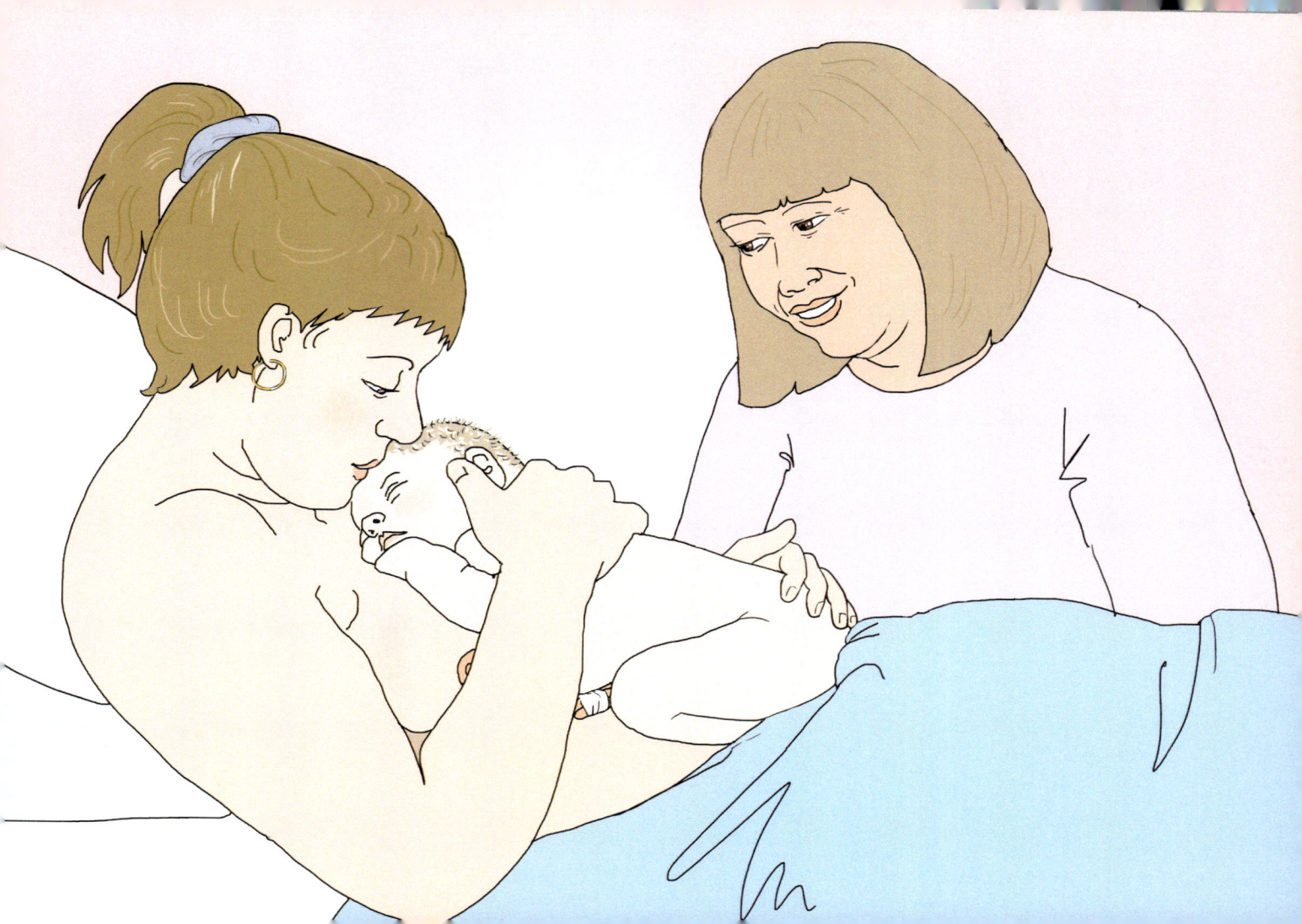

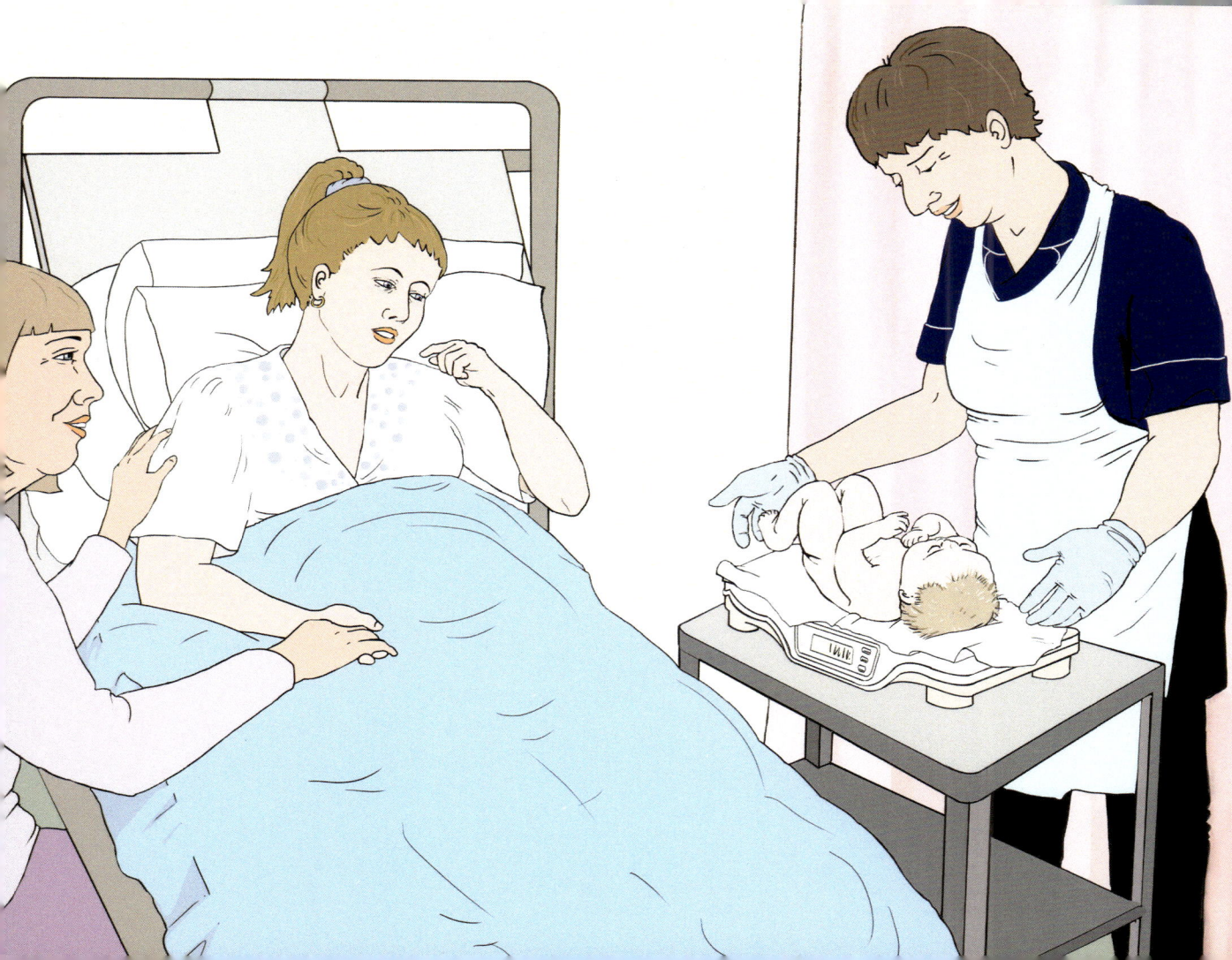

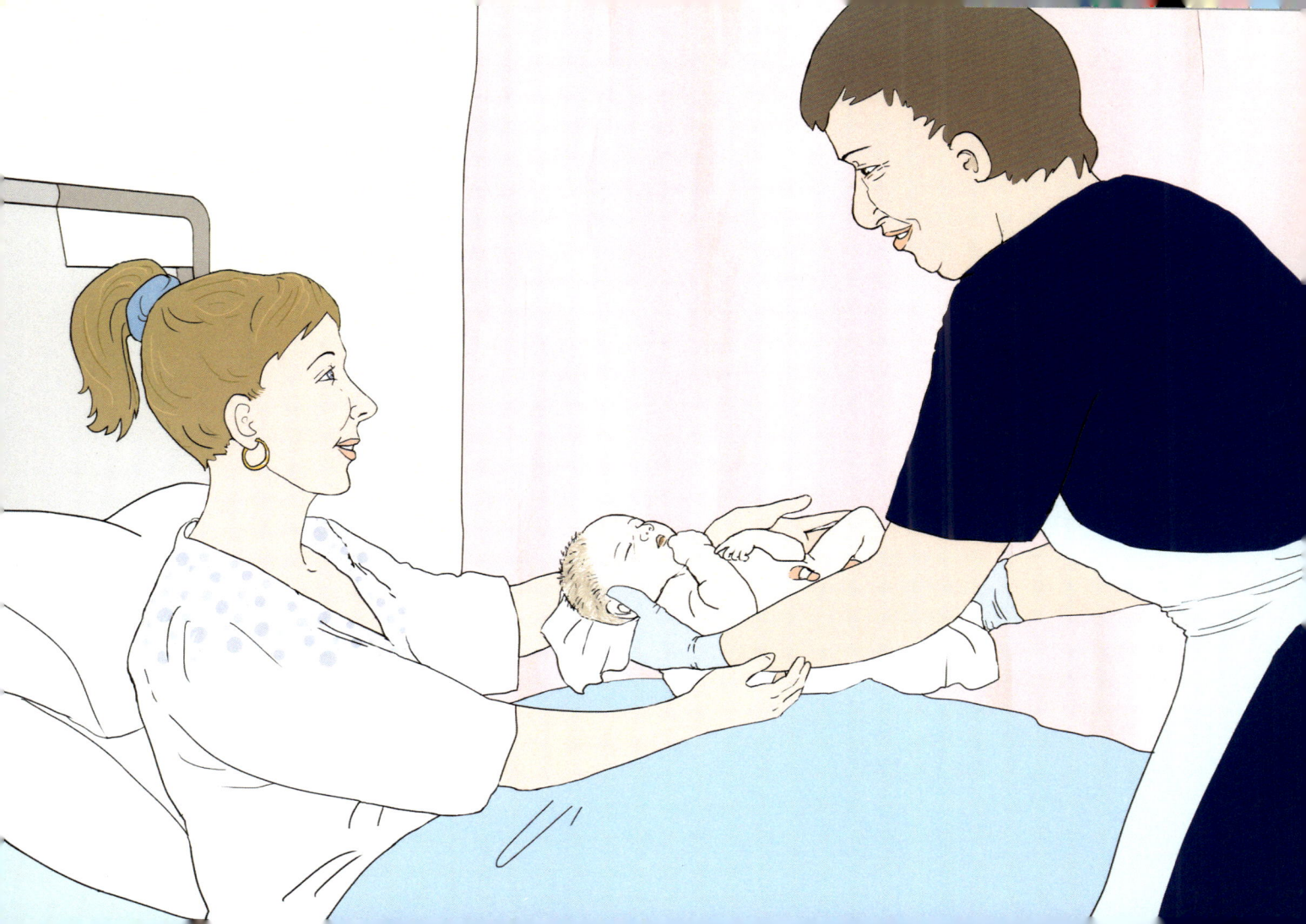

24

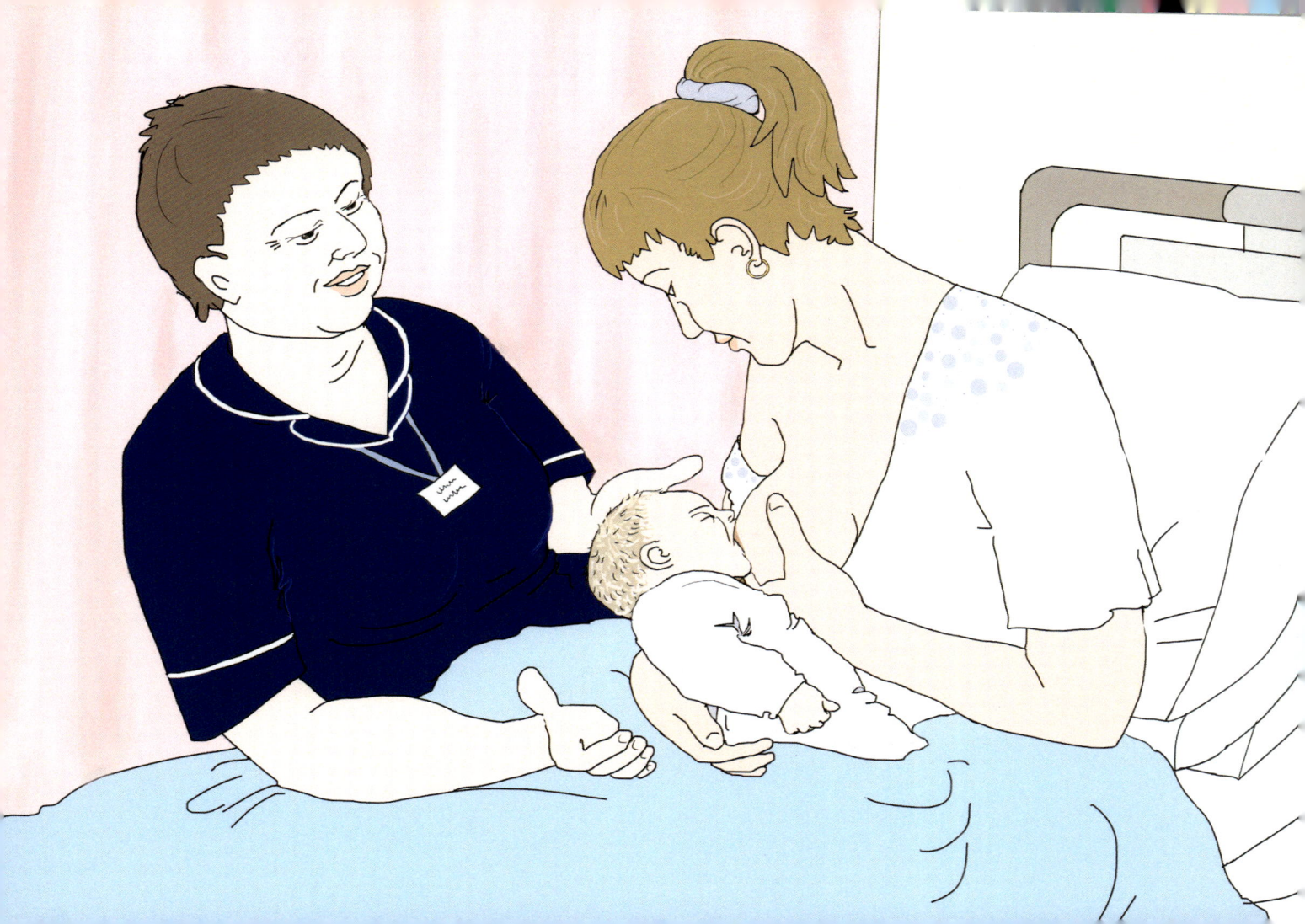

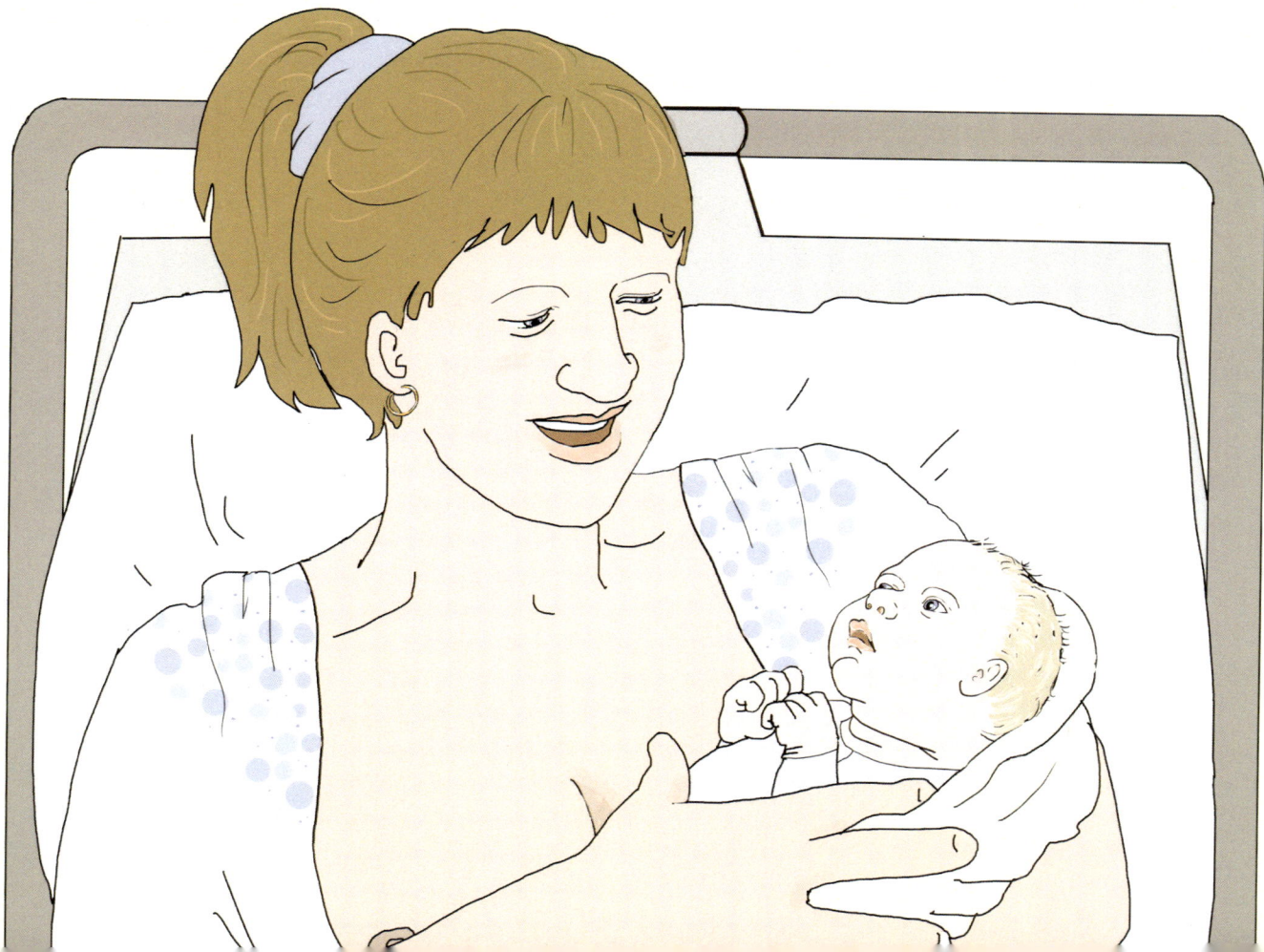

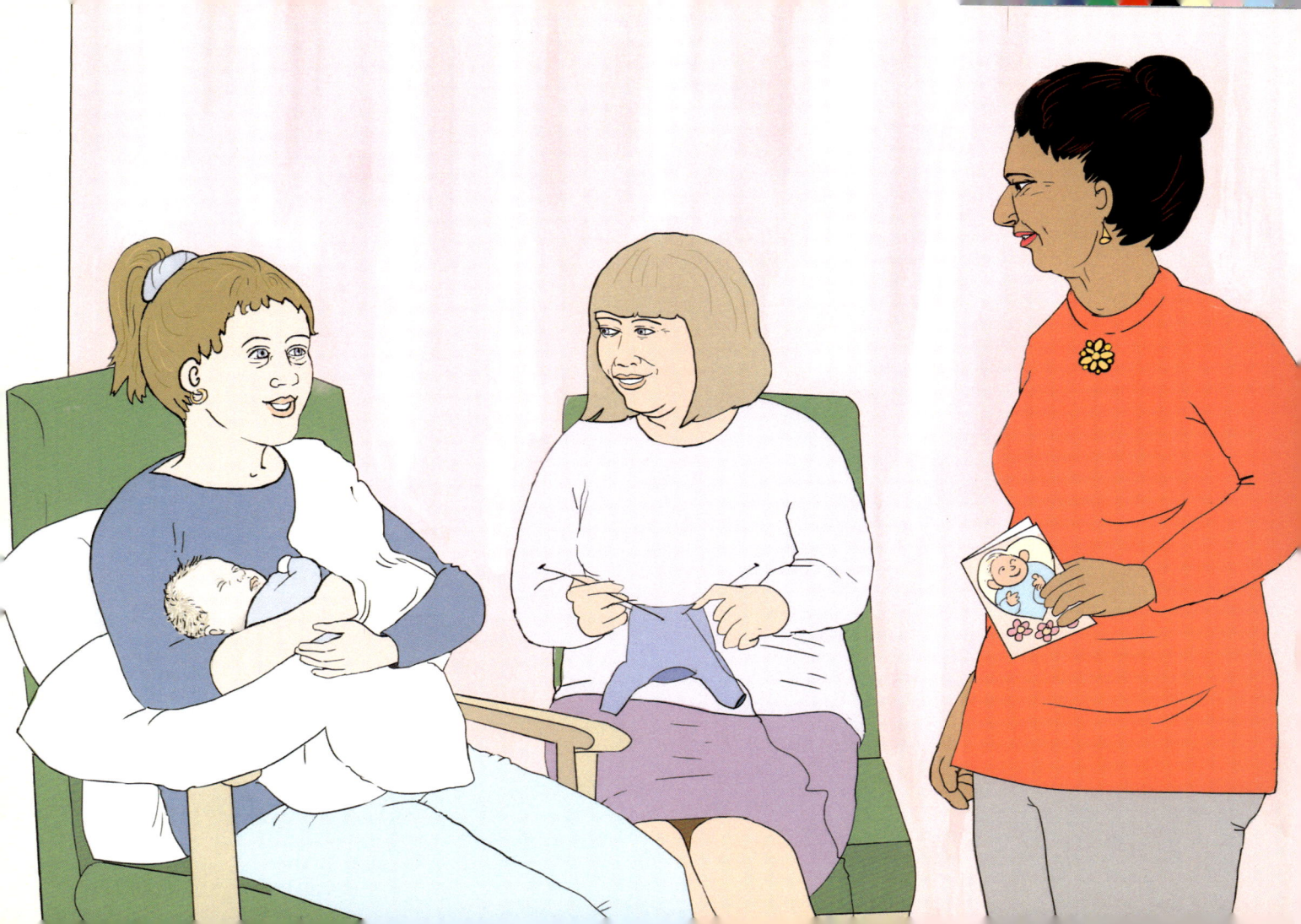

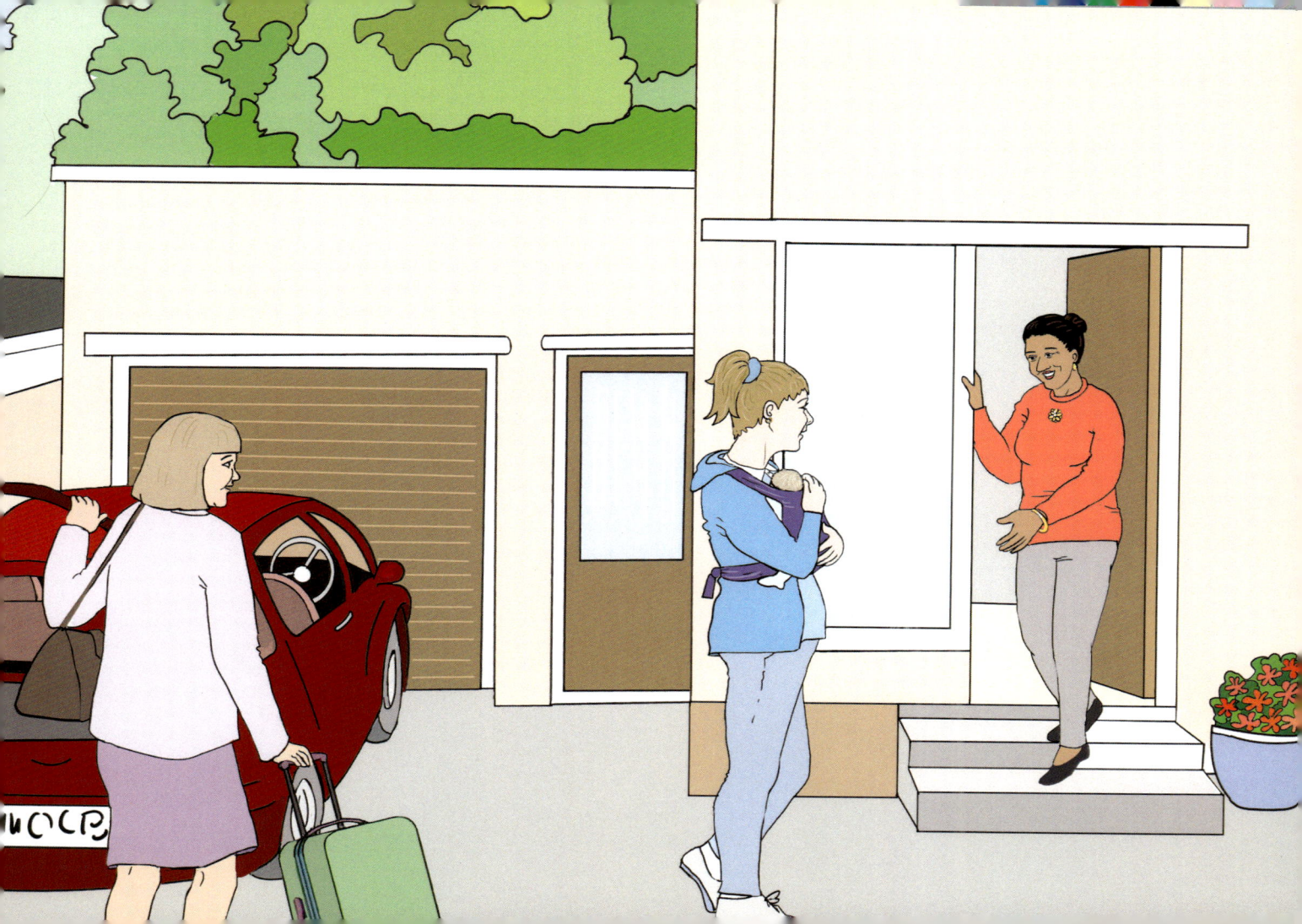

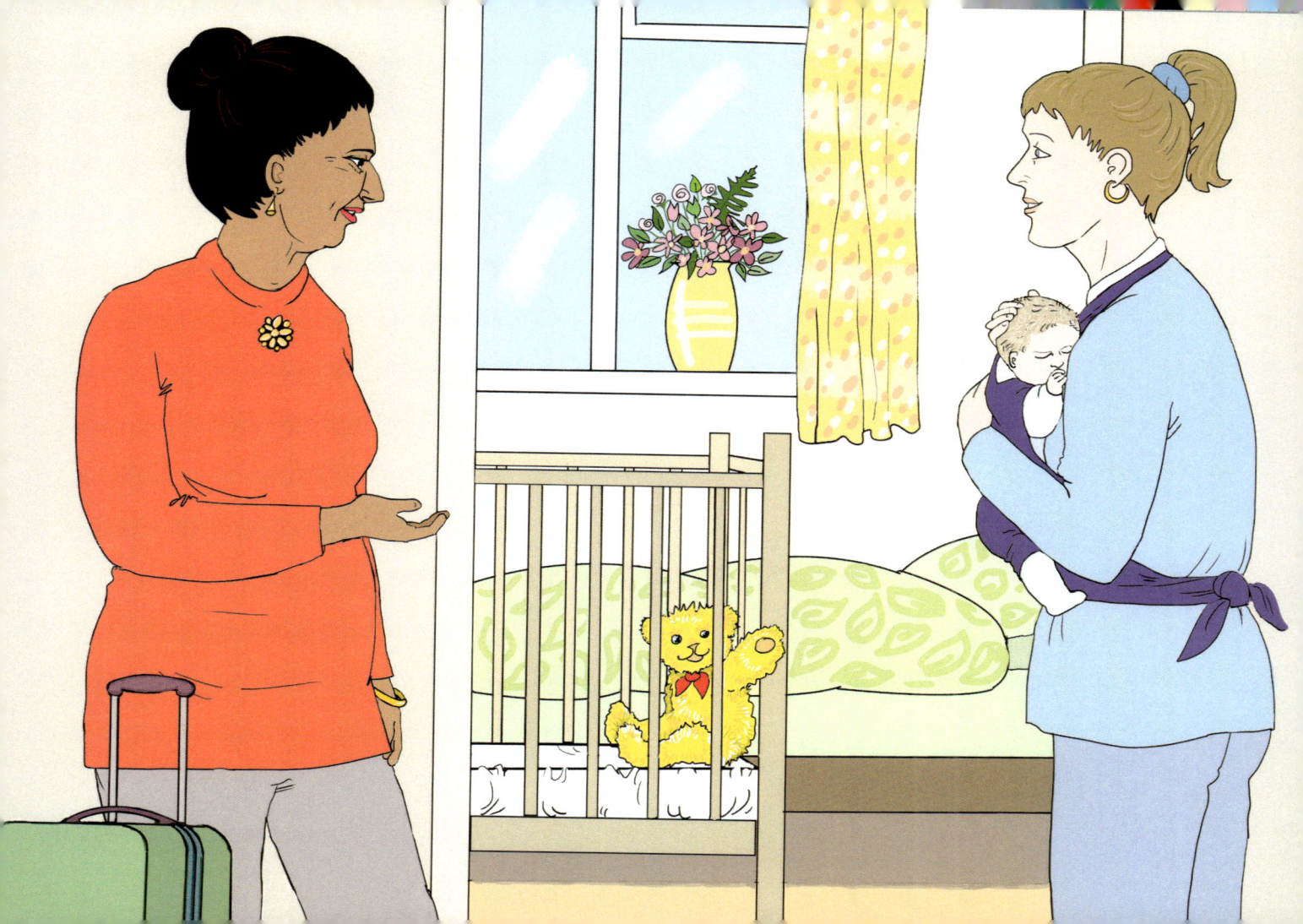

29

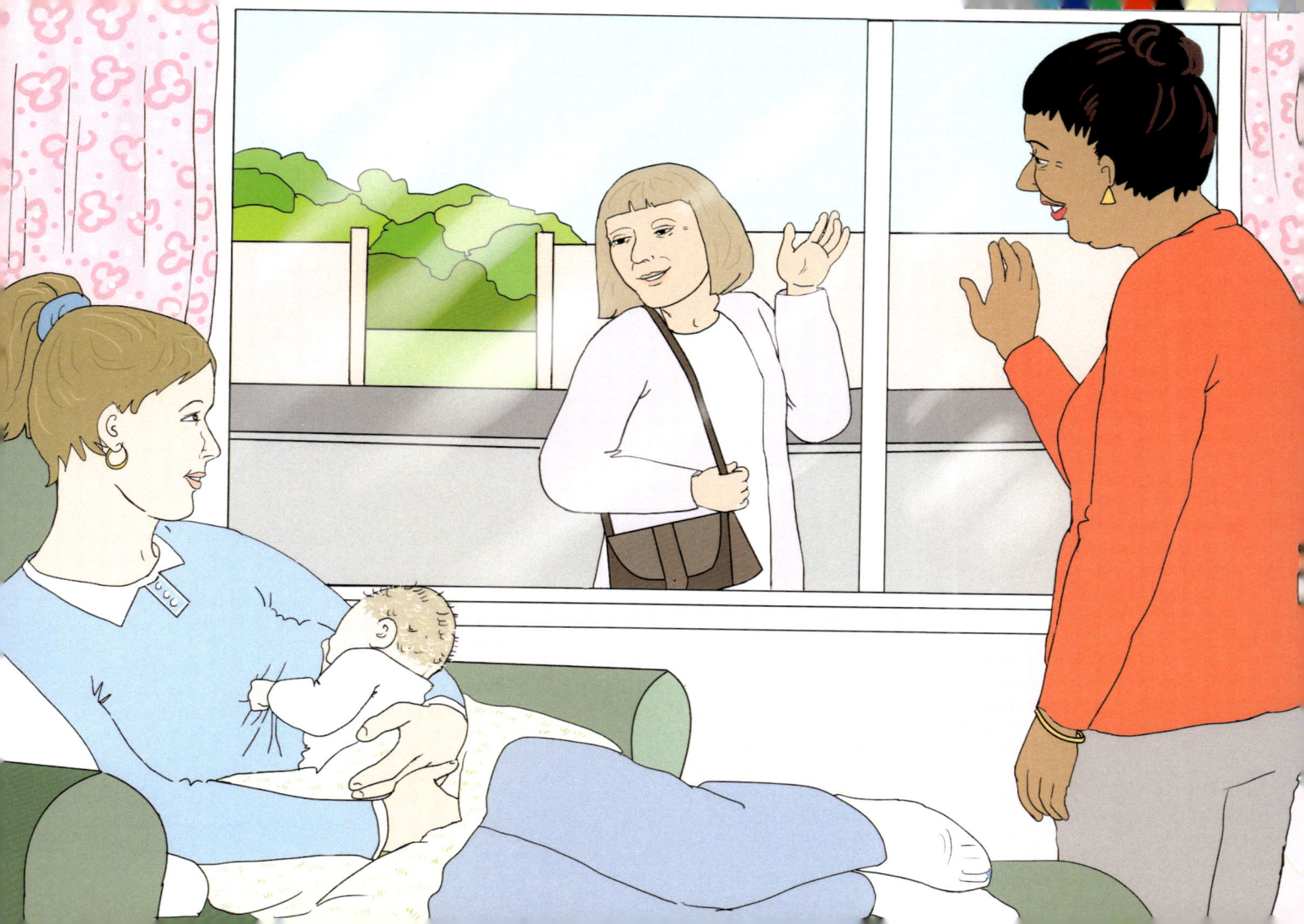

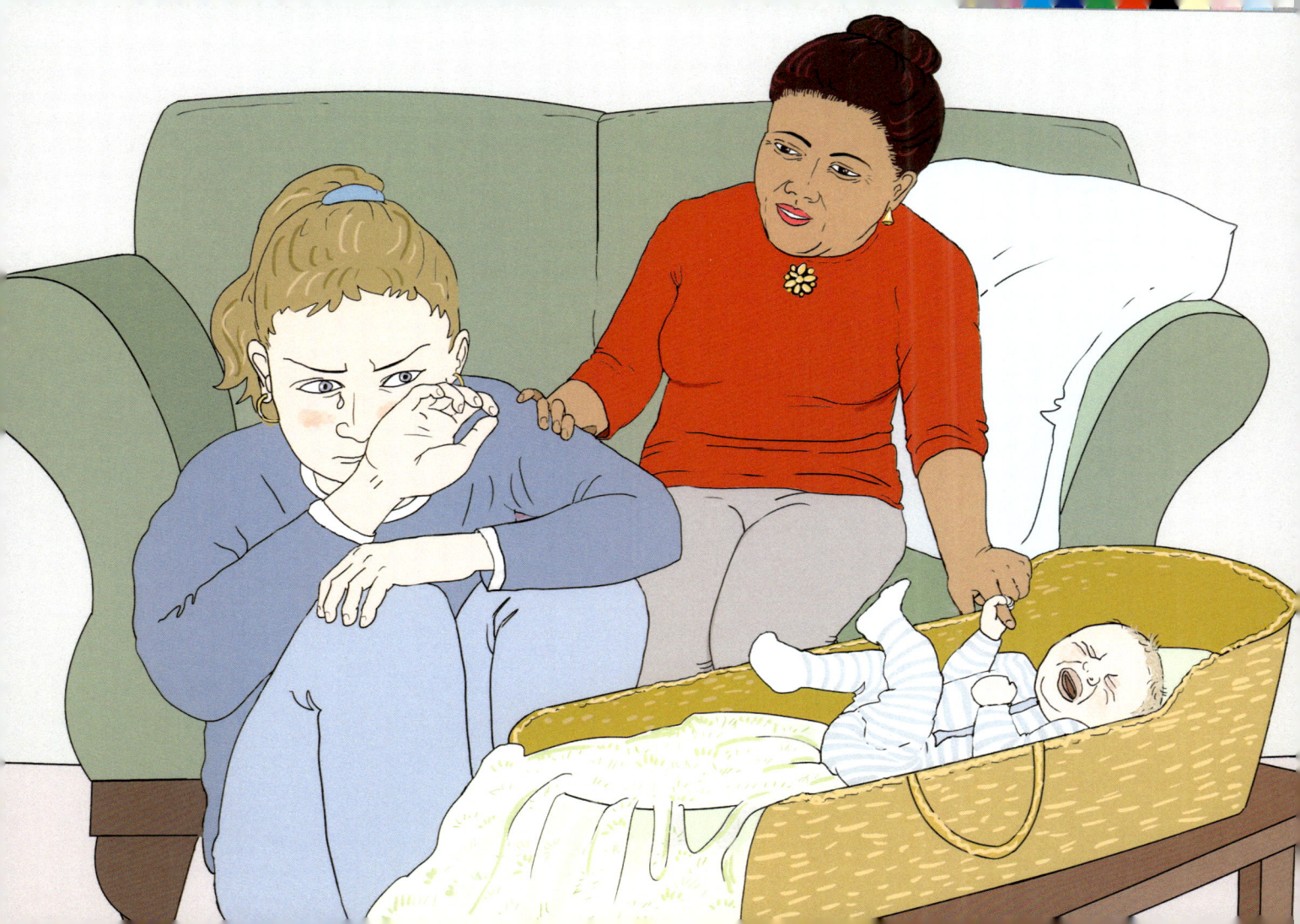

31

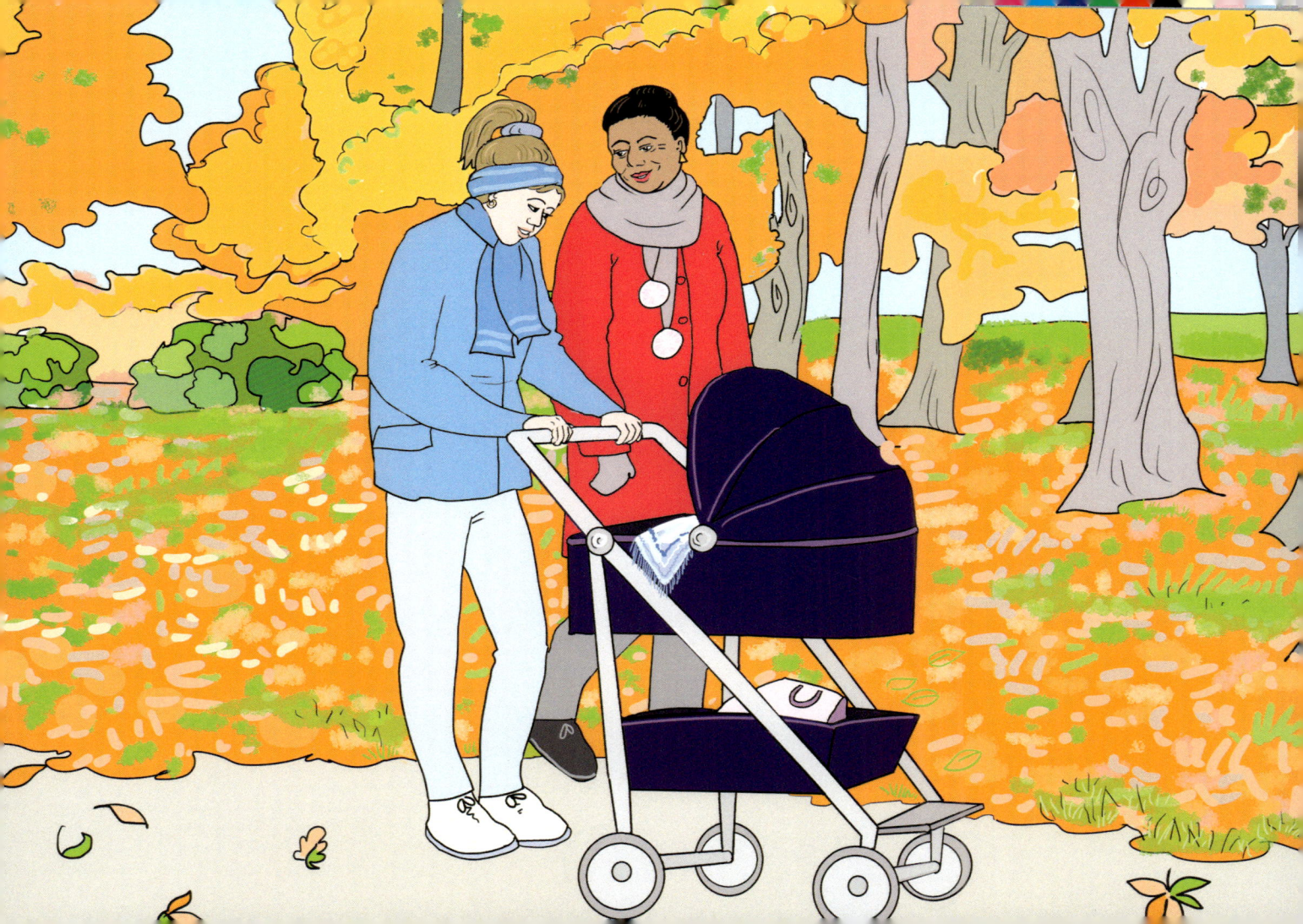

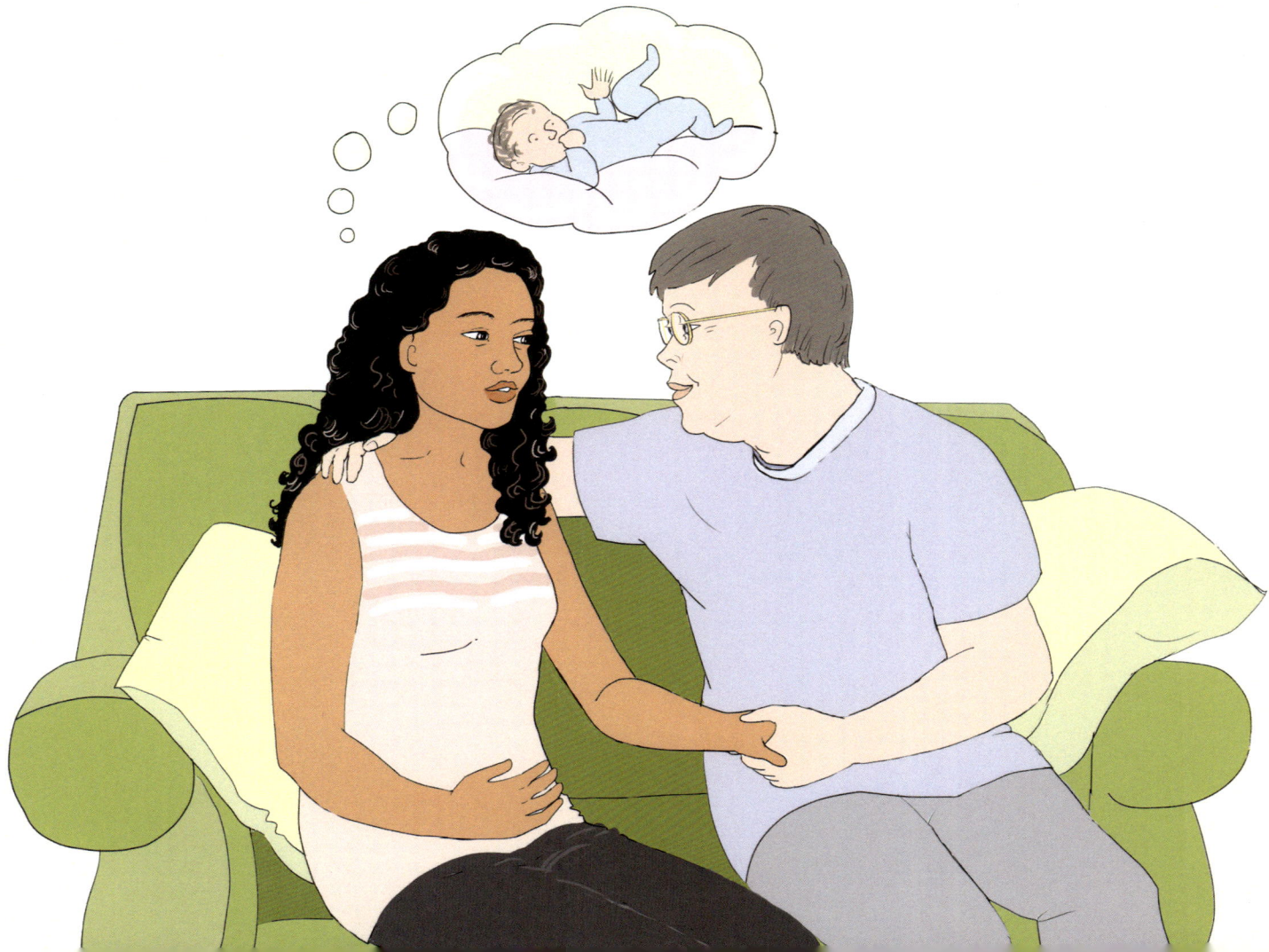

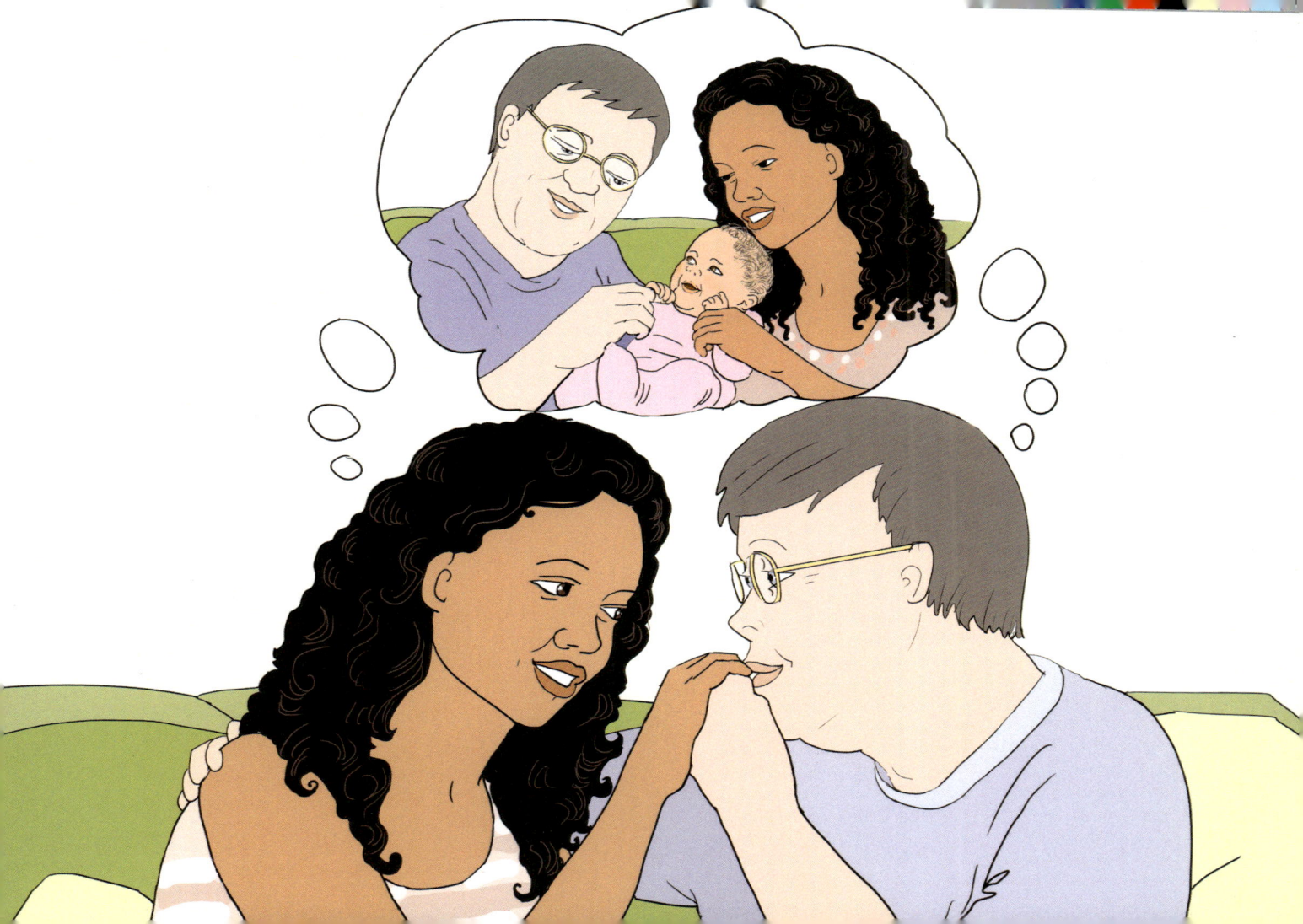

34

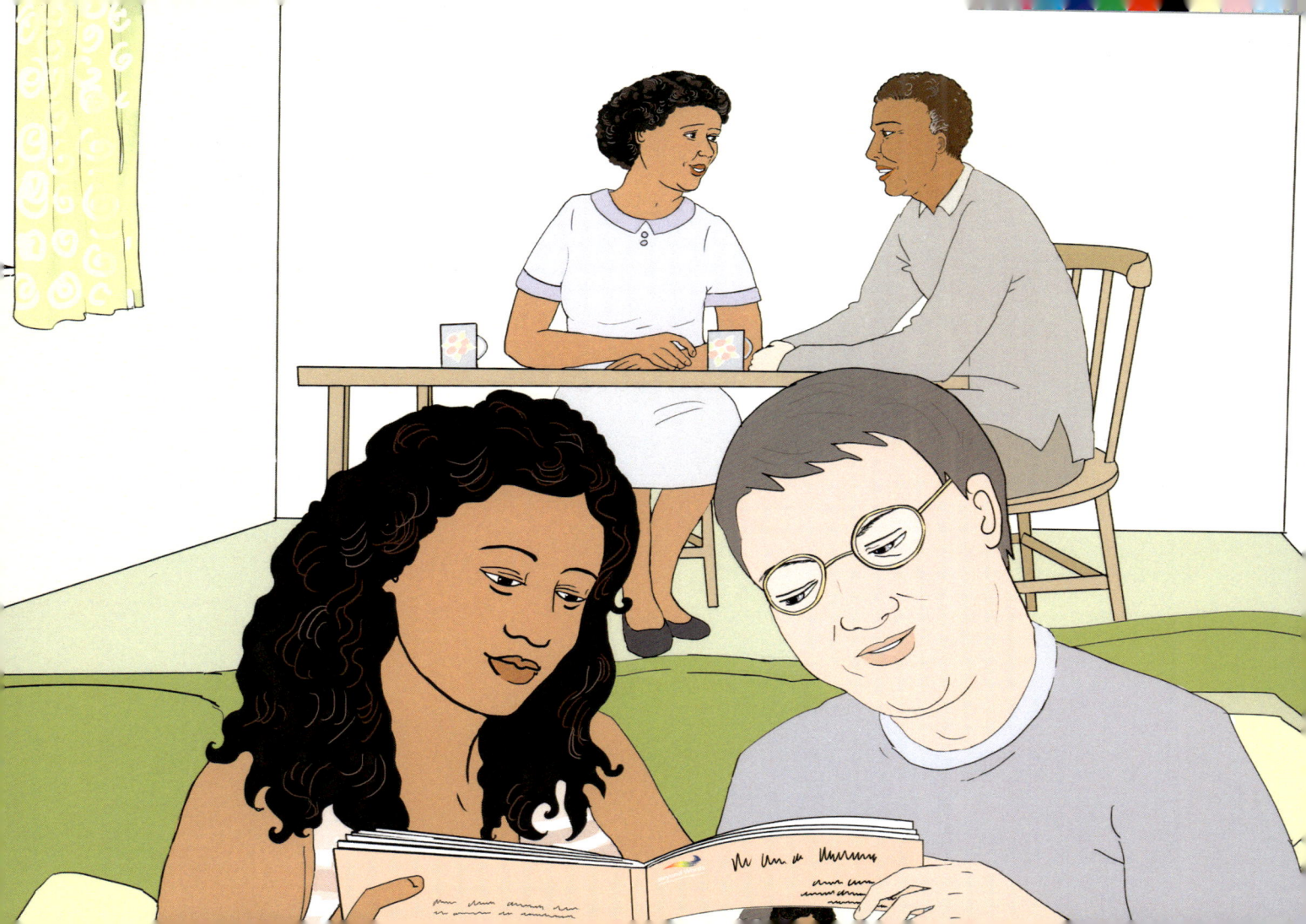

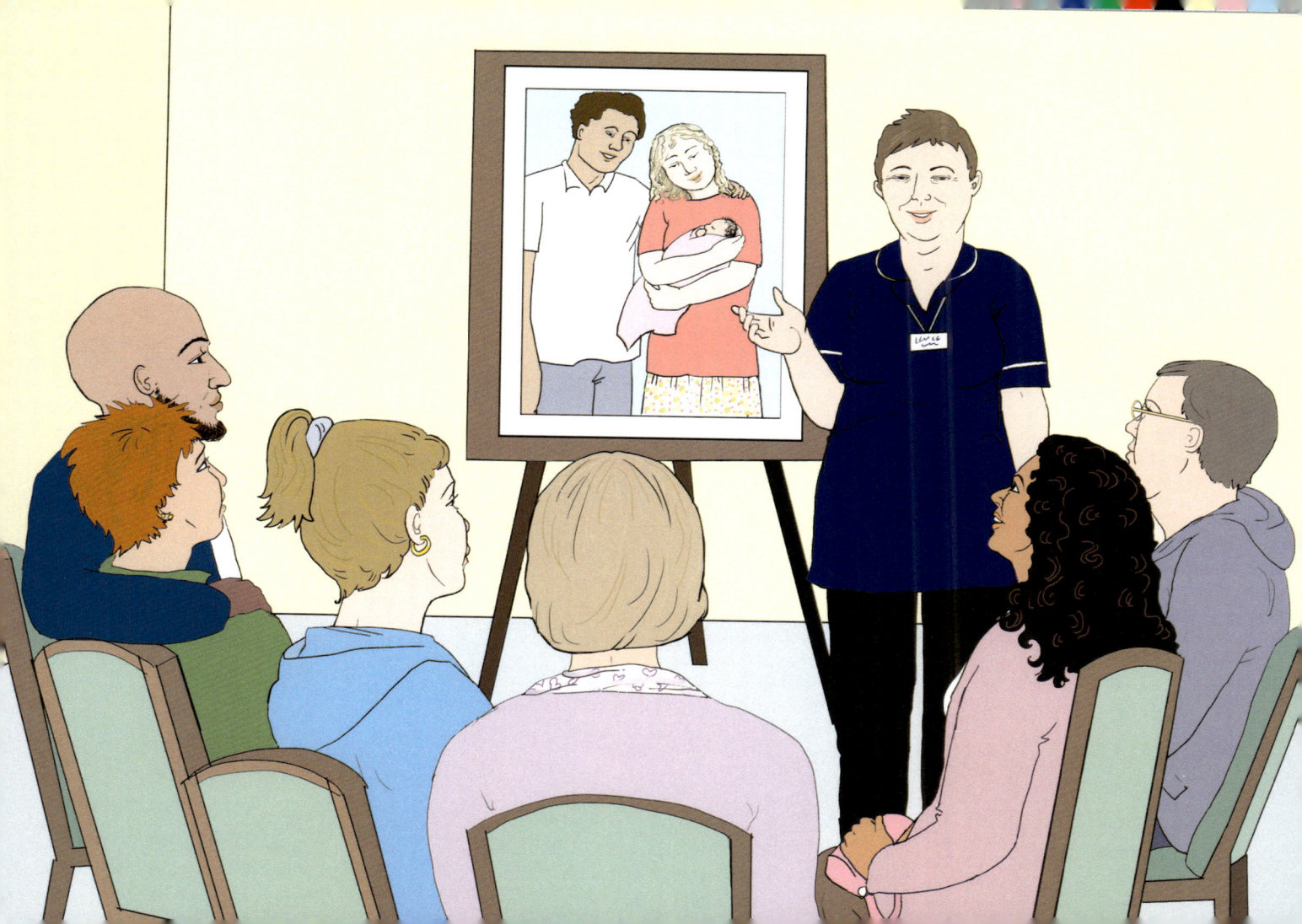

36

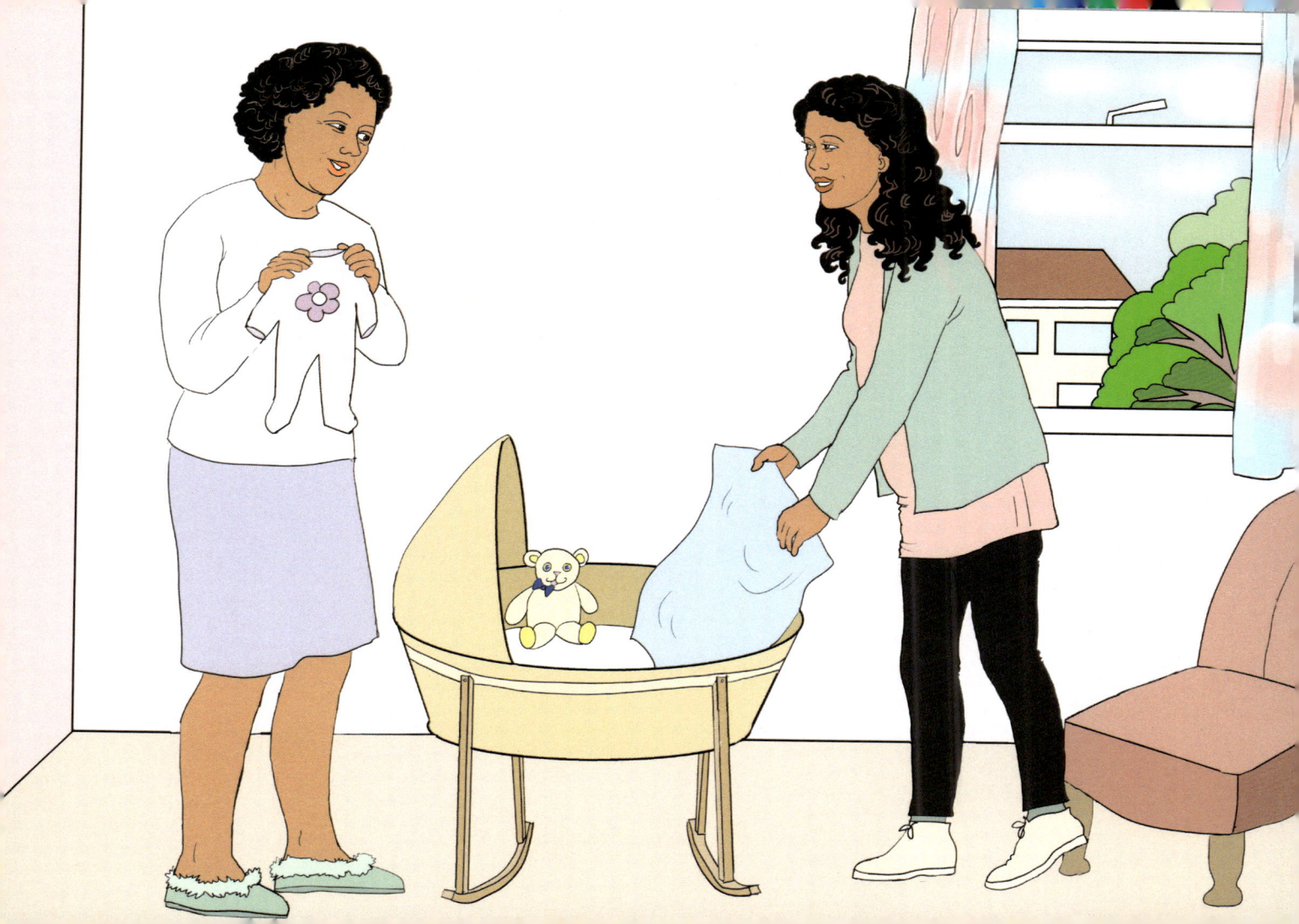

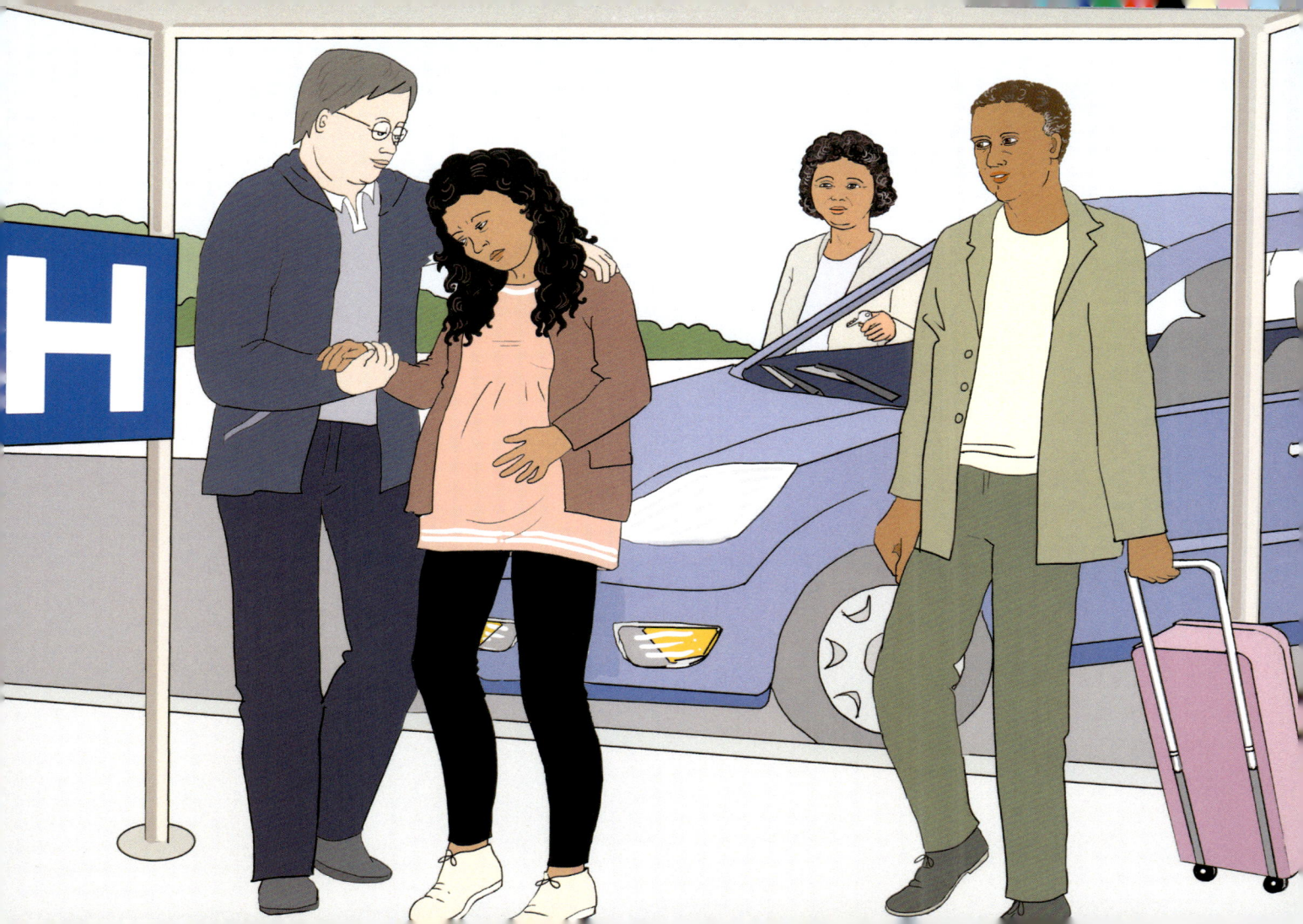

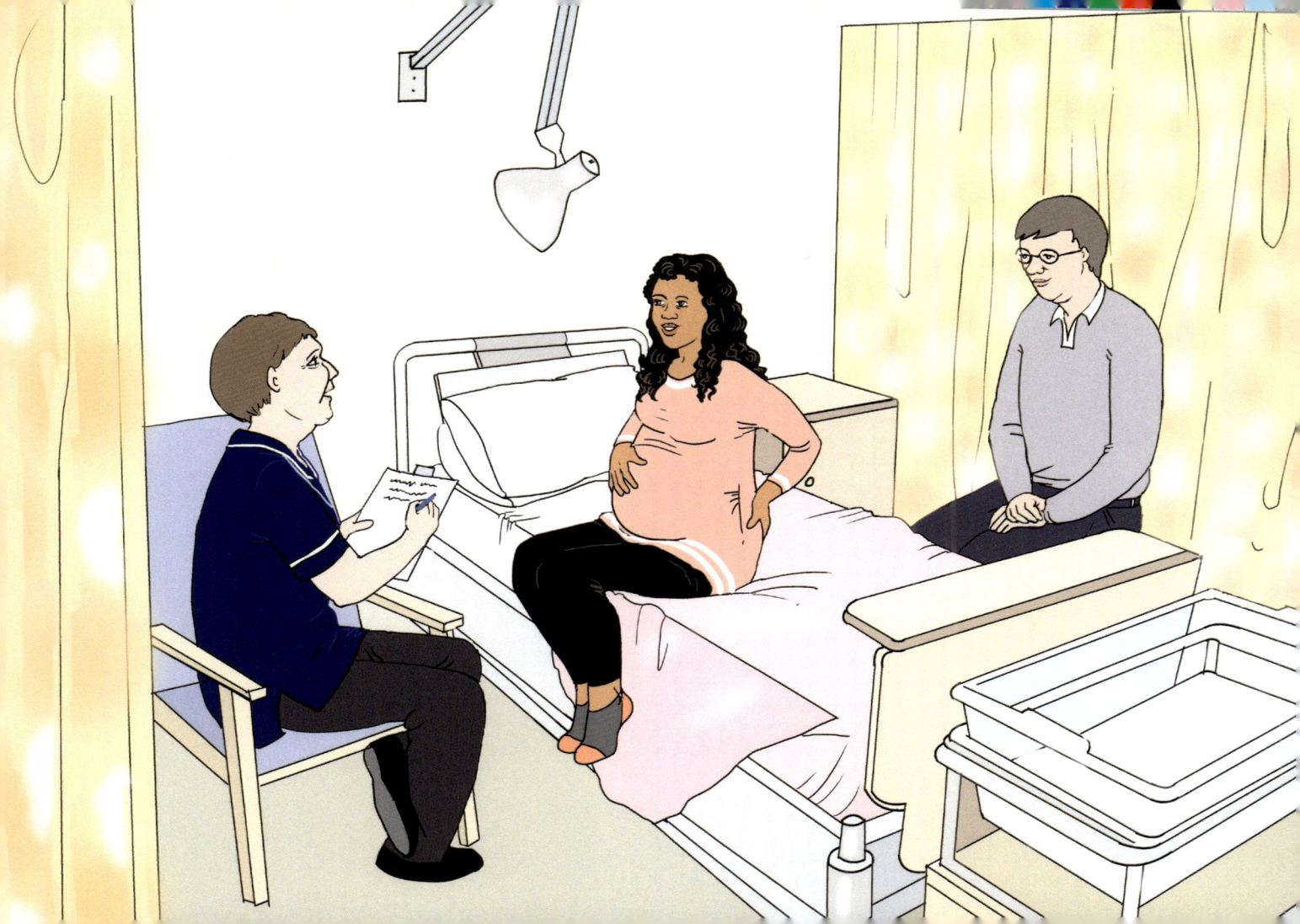

39

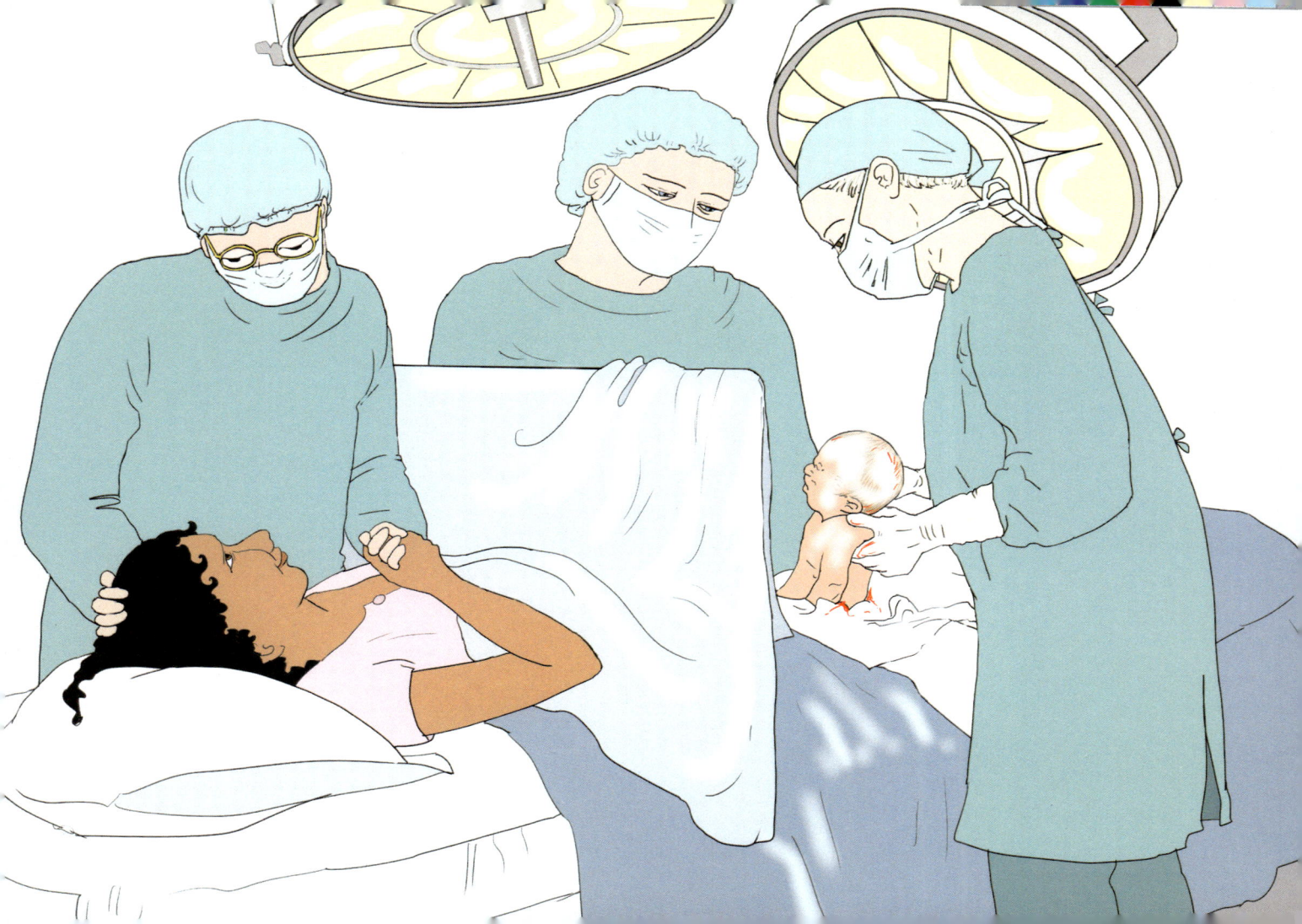

40

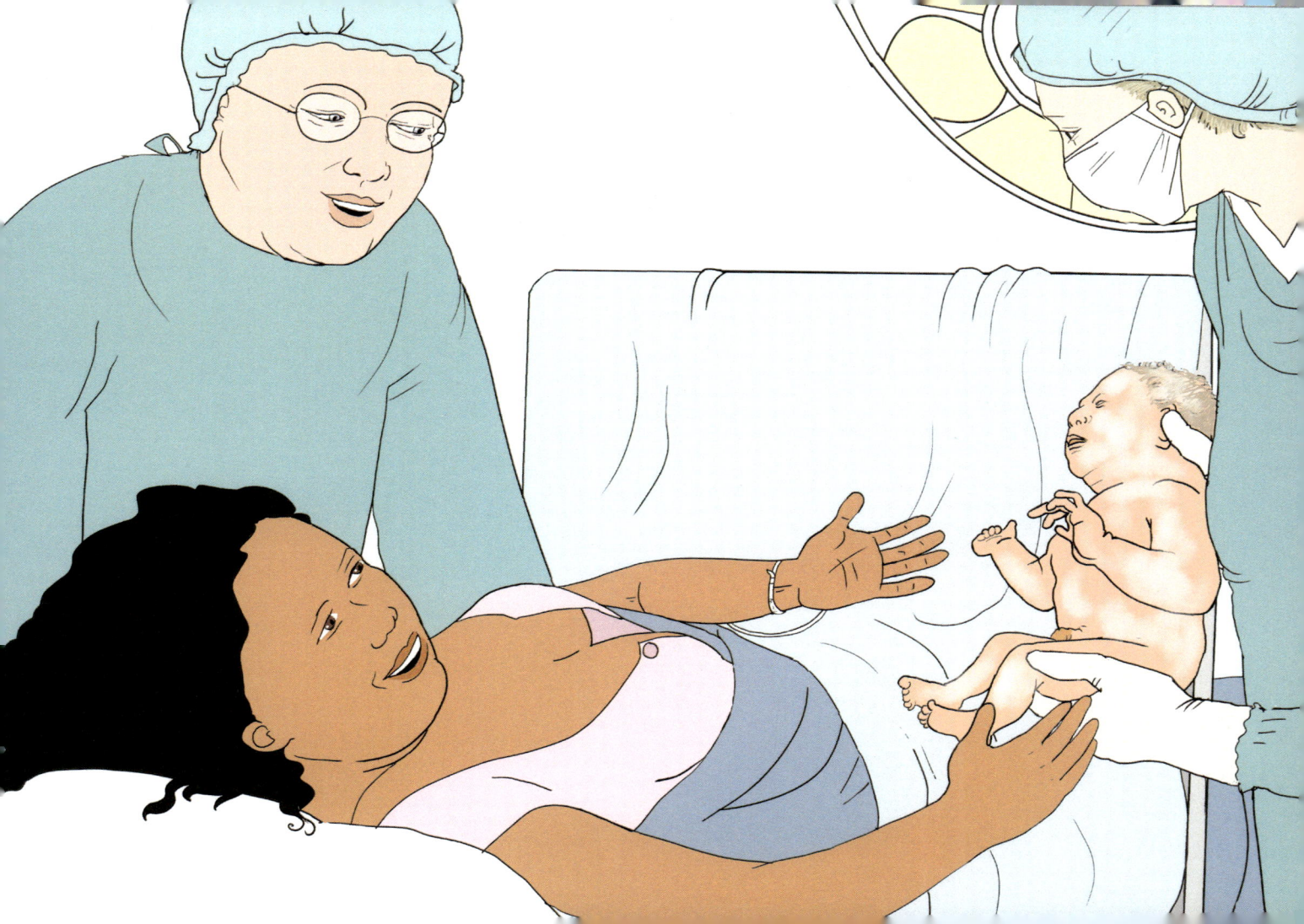

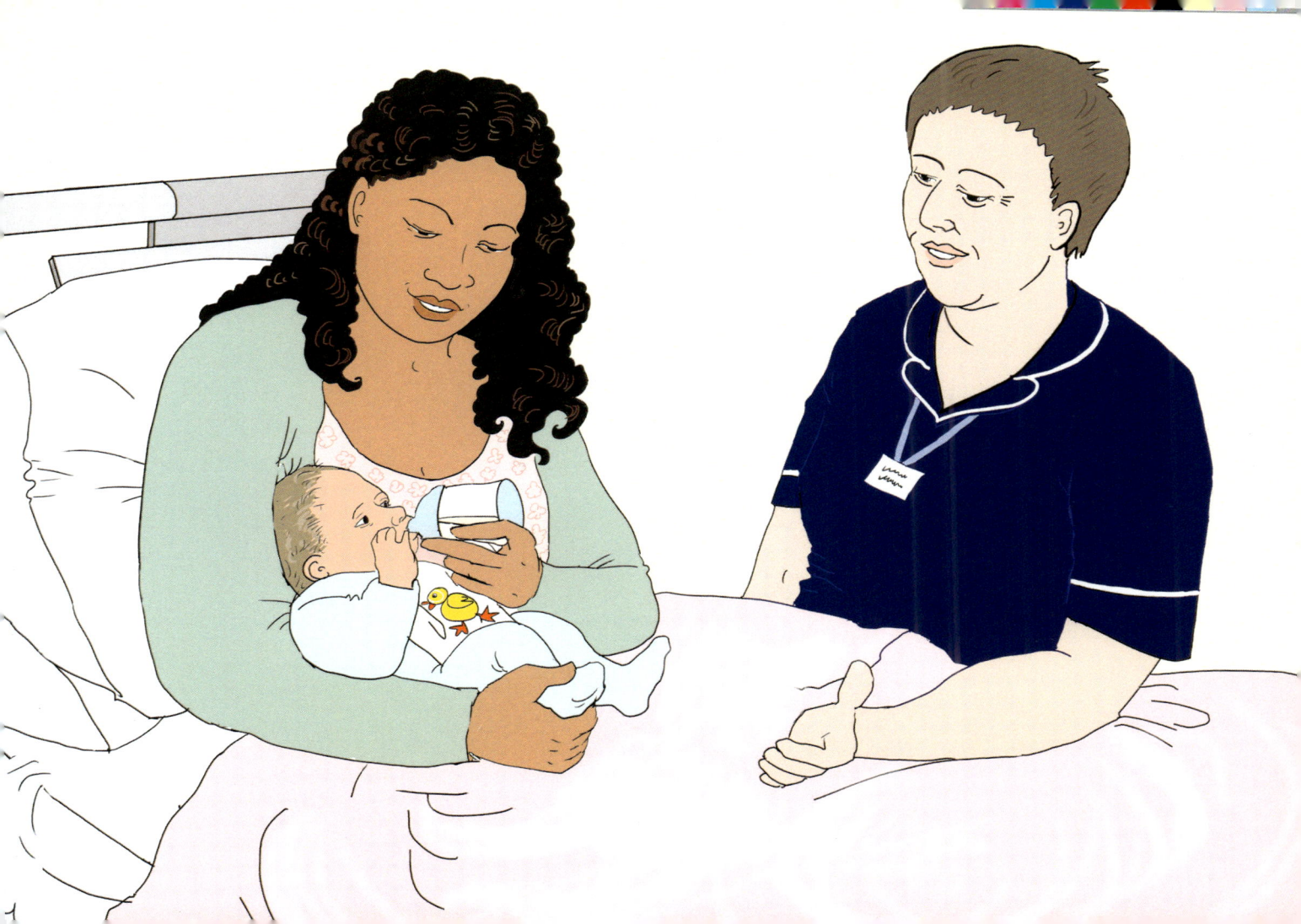

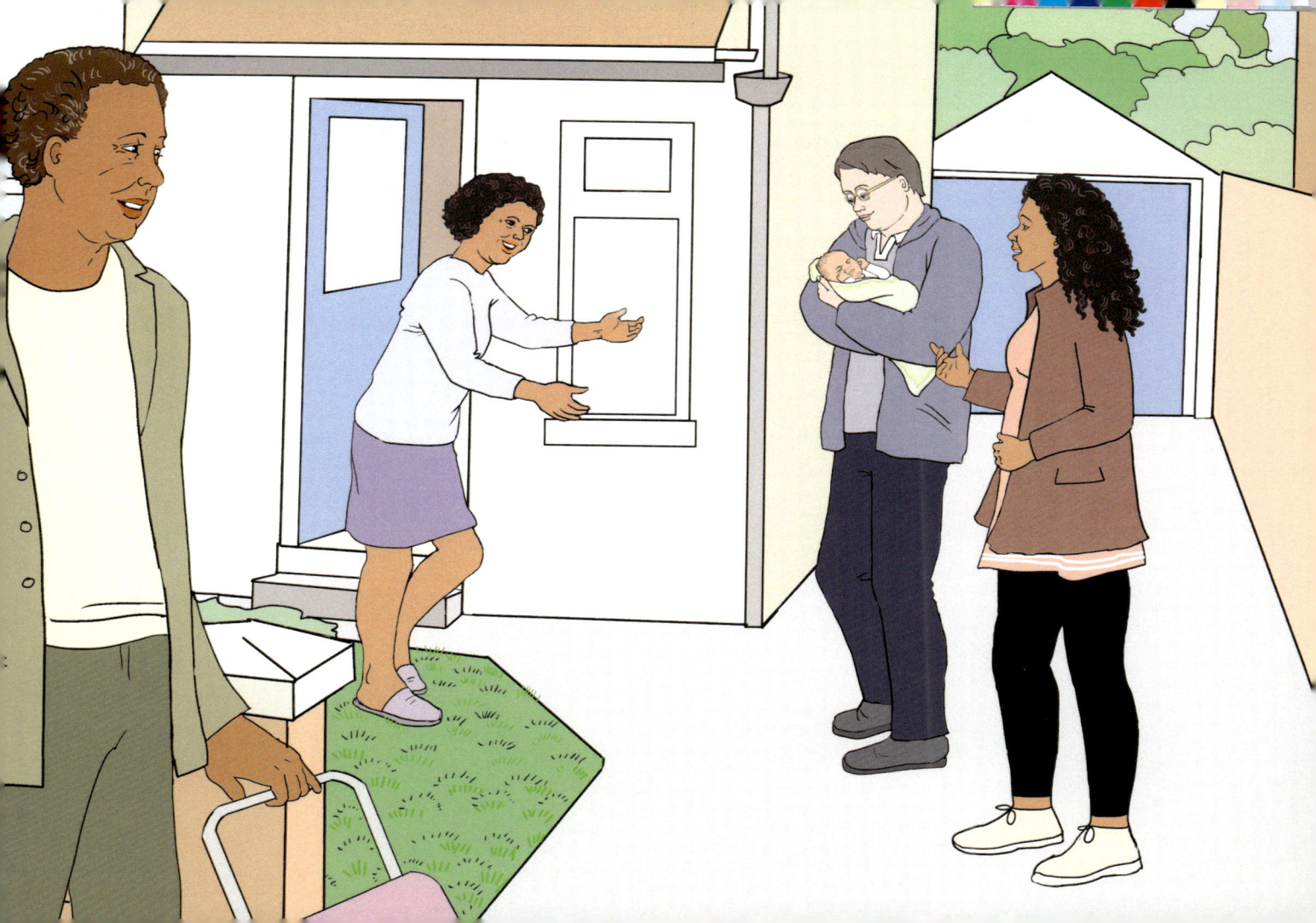

43

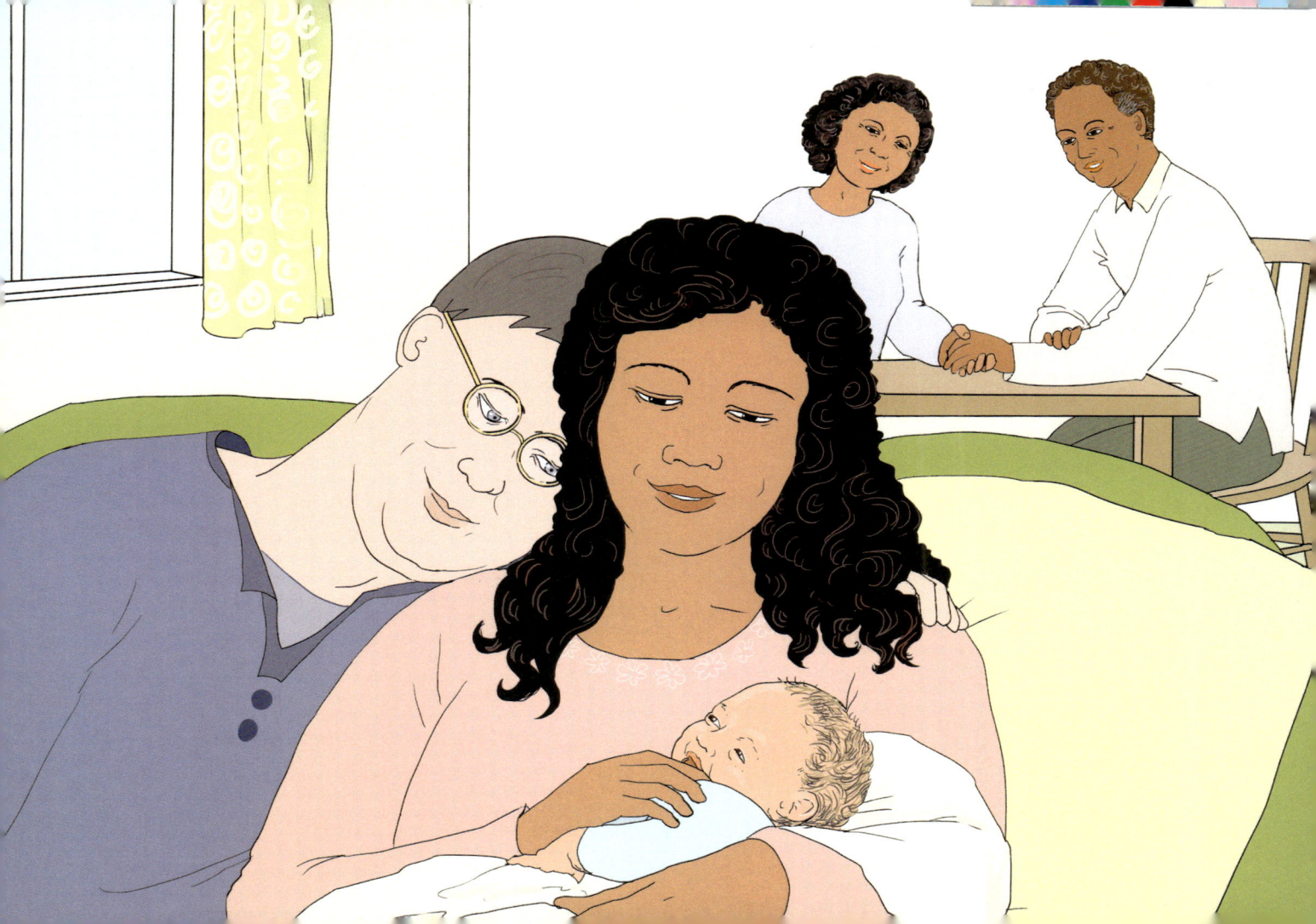

Authors and Artist

Dr Kathryn Hollins supports families, practitioners and communities to create trusting relationships with babies, children and young people, thus building foundations for good lifelong health. She is a Consultant Parent Child & Family Psychiatrist & Psychotherapist. **www.drkathrynhollins.com**

Dr Anna Cox is a Chartered Psychologist and Senior Lecturer in the School of Health Sciences at the University of Surrey. Anna leads the Together Project that has brought together parents with learning disabilities, researchers, and health and social care professionals to co-produce resources to support good maternity care for people with learning disabilities. **www.surrey.ac.uk/togetherproject**

Milli Miller is a parent and a qualified Senior Social Worker and Practice Educator in an Adults' Learning Disabilities Team.

Tessa van der Vord has been a Specialist NHS Mental Health midwife since 2016 and has many years' experience as a midwife in the labour ward, birth centre, maternity inpatient ward and antenatal clinic.

Scott Watkin BEM and his wife, Amanda, both of whom have a learning disability, developed resources with researchers on the Together Project to support good practice in maternity services for parents with learning disabilities. Scott is Head of Engagement at SeeAbility.

Beth Webb is the artist who helped develop the early concept of Books Beyond Words, and since then she has illustrated and helped create 27 titles in the series. Beth is also a children's author and a professional storyteller. Her websites are: **www.bethwebbillustrator.co.uk** and **www.bethwebb.co.uk**

44